CONTENTS

This publication contains the opinions and ideas of the author. Any reliance on the information in this book is at the reader's own discretion.

The author and publisher disclaim all responsibility, loss, or rights personally or otherwise, which is incurred as a consequence, directly or indirectly of the use and application of any contents of this book. They further make no representations or warranties with respect to the accuracy or completeness of the contents of this book.

Any recommendations are made without any guarantee on the part of the author or the publisher.

DEDICATION

This book is dedicated to all the people; young and old, who taught me different tools and techniques on how to stay safe.

Thank you!!!

INTRODUCTION

My beautiful female as you grow older you will discover new things you enjoy doing. Plus, new places you will like to visit. While discovering new things and new places you will encounter new dangers you have to be aware of. With "Girl Did You Know" I hope to empower you with information, tools, and techniques you can use to stay safe while you explore and discover life and all the joy that can comes with it.

Be safe my beautiful female.

INTUITION

My precious female God has blessed you with a wonderful gift called intuition and you should not be afraid to trust it. Your intuition is a tool placed inside of you to warn and protect you from harm and danger. For those of you who still do not understand what intuition is let me explain it to you like this. Your intuition is a feeling that you get in the inside of you letting you know if something is good or bad for you, if a person is a good person or a bad person, and if something is dangerous or if it is safe.

While dating your intuition can be a very helpful tool for you to use. When you are dating and you meet a guy and you get the feeling that he may harm you; trust your intuition and do not go out on a date with him.

When you are meeting new people who are interested in being your friend your intuition can be a helpful tool for you to use. If you get the feeling that the new people you just met is not safe to be around or for you to hang out with; you should trust your intuition and not interact with them. That does not mean you cannot be cordial when you see them; it means you cannot hang out with them as if you all are friends.

If someone ask you to go with them and your intuition is telling you that you should not go because something really bad is going to happen trust your intuition and do not go with them. It is best for you to not go with them and be safe versus going with them and taking a chance on being in an undesirable situation.

My beautiful female what is happening is your spirit is seeing what your physical eyes cannot see. Intuition gives people insight to things that can happen or will happen if the appropriate action is not taken.

Your intuition is there to help protect you so do not ignore it. I would hate for you to ignore your intuition and spend time with someone or doing something that lead to bad things happening to you. Trust your intuition it is there to keep you safe from dangerous people and to keep you from experiencing harm and danger.

HOW TO SAY NO EFFECTIVELY

My beautiful female if you have to tell someone "No" this is how to say "NO" effectively. Make sure when you tell someone "No" that you say "No" very firmly. Do not add any explanation to why you chose to say "No". By giving explanations when you say "No" it can come across as if you are trying to convince yourself of the decision you made. It will also show the person that you do not mean what you say when you say it; all because you have rendered up an explanation for the decision you made.

If the person continues to ask you the same question over and over and over again you can tell him or her very firmly "I Said No" and never address his or her question or request again. If you were to address that person's question or request it will give that person an opportunity to try to change your mind and get you to do something you do not want to do. By not acknowledging the person's question or request after you have told him or her "No" lets that person know that when you say "No" that is what you mean.

DRUGS

My beautiful female; there are a lot of different drugs that people take for recreational purposes (for fun). These drugs are taken for the temporary feeling of pleasure that they give, but what they do not tell you about are all the negative side effects that they have to endure once the high has worn off. Sometime they endure negative side effects during the high.

I want you to be aware of the dangers you will face by taking legal drugs or illegal drugs; or even abusing prescription drugs to get high. What you need to understand is that not all drugs are alike. Some drugs damage the body very gradually and some drugs damage the body very quickly. Also, each drug affects the body differently.

My precious female as you meet new people and make new friends you will find out that some of those individuals use drugs. Those individuals will try to rationalize why they use drugs and why you should use them too.

Here are a few of the excuses people will tell you as to why they use drugs and why you should use drugs too.

- They have medical marijuana so it can't be bad.

- You are supposed to experiment with drugs when you are young.

- If you use it in moderation nothing will happen.

- Drugs ain't bad if you do not use them all the time.

- Ain't nothing good for you anyway; so you might as well go out doing something you enjoy.

- It helps you to relax

- I am bi-polar

- It makes the pain go away

- God made it so it can't be bad.
- You should try everything at least once.
- Marijuana is an herb.
- Ain't nothing wrong with getting high.

There are many more excuses that people will tell you in order to get you to use drugs with them. Just so you know it is ok for you to tell them No.

My beautiful female two people can take the same drug as well as the same amount and both can experience totally different side effects. That is why you should not assume that you will experience the same side effects as other people if you use the same drugs and the same amount of drugs as they did.

I want you to understand that you can become addicted to the drugs that you have used to get high. For those of you who do not know or understand what being addicted to drugs mean let me explain it to you. First of all; there are two types of addictions *Psychological Addiction* and *Physical Addiction.*

When you are psychologically addicted to drugs you crave the feeling that the drug gives you. You will begin to believe that you cannot function unless you are able to feel that feeling once more. When you are physically addicted to drugs your body will physically go through changes if you do not use that drug to get high. Your body will have to have that drug in order for you to function on a day to day basis; even though that drug is totally destroying your body in the process of you using it.

My beautiful female if you decide to stop using that drug or those drugs to get high your body will go through withdrawal and you will experience several symptoms. For those of you who do not know what withdrawal symptoms are let me explain it to you. Withdrawal symptoms are the physical and psychological changes you will experience when you stop using that drug or those drugs to get high.

My precious female your body is a rare and precious jewel and a rare and precious jewel is meant to be cherished and protected from harm and danger by you at all times. By using drugs to get high you are causing harm and damage to your rare and precious

Lora McDuffie

jewel.

CIGARETTES

My beautiful female I want you to know that smoking cigarettes is a very dangerous thing to do. Smoking cigarettes is so dangerous that there is a warning label on every pack of cigarettes in the United States. It is required by law that each and every pack of cigarettes in the United States has a warning label from the Surgeon General listed on it. Some states have ran commercials showing people who have lost limbs, had double bypass heart surgery, trachea surgery, heart attacks, or a stroke from smoking cigarettes.

In some states all businesses are smoke free with the exception of casinos and some bars because of the danger of second hand smoke. For those of you who do not know what second hand smoke is; it is the smoke that the person blows out their mouth and out their nose when they are smoking cigarettes. As you can see smoking cigarettes is very dangerous; as well as breathing in second hand smoke.

My beautiful female cigarettes contain many dangerous chemicals. Some of the chemicals found in cigarettes are:

Nicotine –A deadly and addictive poison

Arsenic – Used in rat poison

Ammonia – Found in floor cleaner

Acetone – Nail polish remover

Formaldehyde – Used to preserve body tissue

Butane – Lighter fluid

Hydrogen Cyanide – Poison used in gas chambers

Cadmium – Found in batteries

Whenever a person inhale cigarette smoke that individual will kill some of the air sacs on their lungs. The air sacs are how the oxygen that a person breathes gets into their bloodstream. If oxygen is unable to get into the bloodstream; the blood cannot flow to the heart and brain like it should. If the blood is unable to flow to the heart and brain; it can cause severe damage to the body. Sometimes the lack of oxygenize blood can lead to brain damage and even death.

For those individuals who have been smoking cigarettes for a long time some of the health issues your body can experience are:

- Heart Disease
- Strokes
- Lung Cancer
- Throat Cancer
- Stomach Cancer
- Bronchitis
- Emphysema (A breakdown of the lung tissue)

These are just a few of the health issues you can experience from smoking cigarettes.

Here are some of the physical changes you can experience if you smoke cigarettes.

- Your teeth becoming discolored
- Your skin wrinkling sooner
- Loosing bone density and that can lead to Osteoporosis
- Your skin turning pale in color
- Developing ulcers on your gums
- Damage to your teeth (tooth decay)
- Discoloration of your fingernails

My beautiful female smoking cigarettes can cause an individual to impair their athletic performance. In other words their athletic skills will not be at their best because their body will not be able to take in the required amount of oxygen it needs simply because the air sacs are damaged because of the cigarette smoking that individual did or was doing. Also, smoking cigarettes can cause that person's body to heal slower than usual if injured. When a smoker decides to stop smoking cigarettes that person will experience withdrawal symptoms. Listed below are some of the withdrawal symptoms a person will experience when that individual stop smoking cigarettes.

- Headaches
- Fatigue
- Dizziness
- Insomnia
- Dry throat
- Coughing
- Gas
- Mood swings
- Dry mouth
- Constipation
- Depression
- Increase in appetite
- Craving cigarettes
- Lack of concentration
- Mental confusion
- Anxiety attack
- Irritability
- Tightening of the chest
- Sore throat
- Runny nose
- Stomach cramps (sometimes very sever cramping)
- Restlessness
- Weight gain

These are just a few of the withdrawal symptoms a smoker can experience once he or she stops smoking cigarettes. Also, the length of time that person will experience withdrawal symptoms will depend on how long the individual has been smoking cigarettes as well as how many.

Another thing you should know is that a female can cause damage to her fallopian tubes by smoking cigarettes. If a female's fallopian tubes are damaged she will have a difficult time getting pregnant or she may become infertile. For those of you who do not know what infertile means it means not being able to have children.

If a *female* do become pregnant and she decides to continue to smoke cigarettes throughout her pregnancy she can cause her baby to experience several undesirable things such as:
- Low birth weight
- Your baby being stillborn (your baby being born dead)
- Lung problems
- Heart problem

My beautiful female you can even experience miscarriages from smoking cigarettes while pregnant. For those of you who do not know what a miscarriage is let me explain it to you. A miscarriage is your body expelling your baby from your body during 1st and 2nd Trimester. During the 1st and 2nd Trimester the baby will not be able to survive independently from their mother body.

Also, I want you to know that there is nothing cool, sweet, sexy, or hot about smoking cigarettes. Smoking cigarettes are is a death sentence to healthy living. It is up to you to decide if smoking cigarettes worth damaging your rare and precious jewel and dying for.

Remember, your body is a rare and precious jewel and a rare and precious jewel should be cherished and protected from harm and danger by you at all times. Smoking cigarettes will cause harm and damage to your rare and precious jewel.

ECSTASY
(3,4 Methylenedioxy – Methamphetamine)

MDMA (*3,4 Methylenedioxy – Methamphetamine*) or Ecstasy as it is normally called is a synthetic drug with hallucinogenic properties in it. My beautiful female you probably heard people say how good Ecstasy is. They will tell you how good they felt when they took Ecstasy. You will hear people say that Ecstasy makes everything better. Colors become brighter and music sounds better. This is why this drug is used at a lot of rave parties as well as glow sticks and glow ropes.

That over whelming since of euphoria that they are feeling is because of the over flow of *Serotonin* in their brain caused by the use of Ecstasy. What they are not telling you about are all the negative side effects you can experience from taking Ecstasy. Listed below are some of the short term side effects a person can experience from taking Ecstasy to get high.

- Hallucinations
- Anxiety
- Chills
- Sweating
- Increase in blood pressure
- Muscle tension
- Paranoia
- Nausea
- Severe dehydration
- Heat exhaustion
- Involuntary teeth grinding

- Blurred vision
- Confusion
- Craving Ecstasy
- Convulsion
- Involuntary jaw clinching
- Increase in body temperature
- Tremors (uncontrollable shaking)
- Pupils dilation
- Difficulty sleeping
- Loss of appetite
- Involuntary pupil movement
- Urinating a lot

Some of the long term side effects a person can experience from taking Ecstasy to get high are:
- Death
- Paranoia
- Depression
- Becoming delusional
- Increase in urination
- Difficulty having an orgasm
- Damage to neurons in the brain that transmit serotonin
- Intracranial bleeding
- Hyperthermia
- Stomach pain
- Convulsion
- Memory Loss
- Confusion
- Drug craving
- Subarachnoid hemorrhaging
- Cramps

I want you to know once the euphoric feeling from the drug has worn off some individuals can feel tremendous sadness or anger. In some cases the person will feel worse than he or she did before that individual took the drug.

You should also know that not all Ecstasy pills are Ecstasy. Sometimes it is PCP, Ketamine, Fentanyl, or any other drug they choose to press into a pill form and call it Ecstasy. You should know that whatever drug that was used to make those fake Ecstasy pills with; you will experience the side effects of that drug.

My beautiful female taking Ecstasy to get high is very dangerous and it can even be deadly.

Some of the other names used for Ecstasy are:

- Adam
- E
- X
- XTC
- Clarity
- Lover's Speed
- Beans
- Love Drug
- E-tarts
- Go
- Hug Drug
- Scooby Snacks
- Euphoria
- Doctor
- Molly
- Eve
- Booty Juice
- Essence
- Chocolate Chip
- Red Devil
- 007's
- Blue Nikes
- Playboys
- Batmans
- MDMA
- California Sunrise
- Cadillac
- Supermans
- X-Files

Lora McDuffie

- Pokemons
- White Diamonds
- Butterflies
- Buddahs
- Promises
- Blue Kisses
- E – Bombs
- Snowball
- Hug
- Roll
- Elephants
- Lovers Special
- Diamonds
- Roca
- Cloud Nine
- Decadence
- Four Leaf Clover
- Dolls
- Doves
- Play Station
- Love Doctor
- Disco Biscuits
- Rave Energy
- Cristal
- Tweety Bird
- Morning Shot
- Blue Nile
- Bermuda Triangle
- Playboy Bunnies
- White Dove
- Blue Dolphin
- Smurf
- Tom and Jerry
- Whiffledust
- Yuppie Psychedelic
- Dennis the Menace

- Egyptian
- Care Bears
- Apples
- 69's

Also, if a person were to mix Ecstasy with other drug that new combination will have its own name too. Listed below are some of those combinations and their names.
- "Candy Flipping" is Ecstasy and LSD
- "Hippie Flipping" is Ecstasy and Magic Mushrooms
- "Kitty Flipping" is Ecstasy and Ketamine
- "Sextasy" is Ecstasy and Viagra
- "Love Flipping" is Ecstasy and Mescaline
- "Elephant Flipping" is Ecstasy and PCP
- "Candy Flipping On A String" is Ecstasy, LSD, and Cocaine
- "Bump Up" is Ecstasy and Cocaine
- "Domex" is Ecstasy and PCP
- "H-Bomb" is Ecstasy and Heroin
- "Chocolate Chip Cookies" is Ecstasy and Heroin
- "Robo Flippping" is Ecstasy and DXM
- "Troll" is Ecstasy and LSD
- "Pikachu" is Ecstasy and PCP
- "Waffle Dust" is Ecstasy and Amphetamine

If a person was to take any of these combinations he or she will experience side effects from each and every drug in that combination.

My beautiful female when you go clubbing (going to the club) it is very important that you do not accept candy from people you do not know. The candy you are accepting could be Ecstasy. Once you have taken this drug you will do things you normally will not do. You will be conscious of what you are doing, but you will not be able to help yourself because the desire will be too strong.

This drug will give you the desire to touch people as well as be touched. Due to the over whelming desire to touch and to be touched it can lead to you having sex with people you do not know. Plus, people who you will normally not have sex with.

To make matters worse you may even contract Human Immunodeficiency Virus (HIV) or a different Sexually Transmitted Disease (STD) because of your promiscuous sexual behavior. In addition to contracting a STD you may become pregnant. Plus, you may have a difficult time trying to figure out who the father of your child is because of your promiscuous sexual behavior.

My precious female it is very important that you know the dangers of taking Ecstasy.

Remember, your body is a rare and precious jewel and a rare and precious jewel should be cherished and protected from harm and danger at all times by you. Using Ecstasy to get high is not how you cherish and protect you will your rare and precious jewel.

KETAMINE

My beautiful female; for those of you who do not know what Ketamine is let me tell you. Ketamine is an anesthetic used by veterinarians on animals in order to operate on them. It has also been used in dentistry and in pediatrics burn cases. This drug is a dissociative anesthetic.

Some of the short term side effects a person can experience from using a low dose of Ketamine to get high are:
- Confusion
- Vomiting
- Sweating
- Blurred vision
- Motor skills are impaired
- Constricted pupils
- Dissociation of body
- Hallucination
- Distorted vision
- No concept of time
- Difficulty concentrating
- Disorganized thoughts
- Slurred Speech
- Increase in blood pressure
- Increase in heart rate
- Nausea
- Numbness in your legs
- Numbness in your arms
- Distorted perception of sounds
- Distorted perception of sight
- No concept of space

- Impaired judgment
- Lack of coordination

Some of the long term side effects a person can experience from taking a low dosage of Ketamine to get high are:
- Flashbacks (reliving previous experiences)
- Difficulty remembering things
- Difficulty focusing
- Difficulty learning new things
- Illogical thinking
- Depression
- Personality changes
- Mood swings
- A tolerance to the drug Ketamine

If an individual were to take a high dosage of Ketamine to get high that person can experience some of the side effects listed below.
- Sliding into a coma
- Panic attacks
- Paranoia
- Muscle tension
- Amnesia
- Drowsiness
- Erratic behavior
- Convulsions
- Hostile behavior
- Increase in body temperature
- Bizarre behavior
- Fever
- Depression
- Delirium
- Potentially fatal respiratory problems

Ketamine comes in several different forms: powder, pills, and liquid. Ketamine in its liquid form is clear, odorless, and tasteless; it is being used as a date rape drug. This is why you should never accept drinks from strangers. Or drink a drink that you have left unattended especially if you are in a club, at a bar, or at a party. You should not drink that drink because your drink could have been spiked with Ketamine.

If you drink a drink that has been spiked with Ketamine it will impair your judgment. It will cause you to be incoherent to what is going on to you and around you. If a large dosage of Ketamine was place in your drink you can become immobile. If your judgment is impaired or you are incapable of movement it makes it easier for the person who spiked your drink to rape you, rob you, abduct you, or murder you. Or the person who spiked your drink can do all four things to you. I want you to know that any drink you drink can be spiked with Ketamine. That includes water, soda, juice, milk, and alco.

My beautiful young female listed below are some of the other names used for Ketamine.

- Cat Valium
- Honey Oil
- Jet
- Purple
- Special K
- Super Acid
- Keller
- Special La Coke
- Kit – Kat
- Cat Killer
- Green
- Ket
- Vitamin K
- Blind Squid
- Kellys days

Also if a person was to mix Ketamine with other drugs that new combination will have its own name too. Listed below are some of those combinations and their names.

- "Kittie Flippin" is Ketamine and Ecstasy
- "Meow" is Ketamine and Mephedrome
- "Green" is Ketamine, PCP, and Marijuana

You should know that if anyone was to take any of these combinations that person will experience side effects from each and every drug in that combination.

Remember, your body is a rare and precious jewel and a rare and precious jewel should be cherished and protected from harm and danger at all times by you. Using Ketamine to get high is not an act of cherishing and protecting to your rare and precious jewel.

HEROIN
(Diacetylmorphine)

Heroin (*Diacetylmorphine*) is a highly addictive drug made from the opium poppy plant.

My beautiful female you need to know that this drug is extremely addictive and deadly. The addiction to Heroin will not happen gradually it will happen very fast. Sometimes as fast as the end of your first time using it. If a person was to use Heroin and the purity level was very higher that person could die after their first use. I cannot stress to you how addictive Heroin is. I can only tell you that it is very addictive. So please do not ever try it.

If you were to use Heroin to get high some of the short term side effects you will endure are:

- Muscle weakness
- Constipation
- Vomiting
- Dry mouth
- Your arms become very heavy
- Your legs become very heavy
- Itching
- Slurred speech
- Nausea
- You will alternate between being alert to drowsy; this is called "*On The Nod*"
- Dilated pupils
- Droopy eyelids
- Respiratory problems

- Weight loss
- Chills
- Loss of appetite

Some of the long term side effects that you can experience from using Heroin to get high are:
- Collapsed Veins
- Infection of the heart lining
- Infection of the heart valves
- Liver disease
- Addiction
- Pneumonia
- Abscesses
- Malnutrition
- Cellulitis

My precious female once a person start taking Heroin it is very hard for them to stop because the withdrawal symptoms are extremely painful. For those of you who do not know what withdrawal symptoms are let me explain it to you. Withdrawal symptoms are the different physical and psychological changes the body will go through if a person stops using Heroin to get high.

Listed below are some of the painful withdrawal symptoms a person can experience when that person stop using Heroin to get high.
- Muscle pain
- Bone pain
- Vomiting
- Aching body
- Diarrhea
- Kicking movements
- Tremors
- Panic attack
- Cold flashes
- Insomnia
- Drug craving
- Goose bumps

- Anxiety
- Irritability
- Restlessness
- Weakness
- Sweating
- Loss of appetite
- Chills
- Flu like symptoms
- Sneezing
- Runny nose
- Stomach cramps

These are a few of the withdrawal symptoms a person can experience once he or she stops using Heroin to get high. Also, the length of time that person will experience withdrawal symptoms will depend on how long that person been using Heroin to get high as well as the amount of Heroin that was being used.

Since the withdrawal symptoms are so painful Heroin users will take more and more Heroin in order to stop the pain. Which means the amount of Heroin the Heroin addict take will have to increase in order to give him or her "the rush" (euphoric feeling) he or she needs in order to not feel the pain. As you can see this is just a vicious cycle that can lead to a Heroin addict spending hundreds and hundreds and hundreds of dollars to support their Heroin habit.

The need for a Heroin addict to take Heroin can cause that person to overdosing on Heroin. For those of you who do not know what overdosing is let me explain it to you. When a person overdoes on drugs that person has taken an amount that their heart is unable to handle. Because their heart is unable to handle the drugs he or she has taken it will stop beating. In some cases the heart will explode in the person's chest cavity. Once their heart stopped beating or exploded in their chest cavity he or she will die.

My lovely female you need to know that a Heroin Addict is a very good candidate for contracting the Human Immunodeficiency Virus – (HIV) and the Hepatitis Virus. If a Heroin

Addict uses a syringe that has blood infected with the Human Immunodeficiency Virus inside it the contaminated blood will be transferred into their bloodstream. Once the contaminated blood is in their blood stream their blood will become contaminated with the Human Immunodeficiency Virus. Just so you know once your blood becomes infected with the HIV Virus it will destroy your immune system. Once your immune system is completely destroyed by the HIV Virus you will develop AIDS (Acquired Immune Deficiency Syndrome). Now that your body is infected with the AIDS Virus your body will deteriorate at an alarming rate. That deterioration will eventually lead to your death.

If a Heroin Addict uses a syringe that has blood infected with the Hepatitis Virus inside it the contaminated blood will be transferred into their bloodstream. Once the contaminated blood is in in their bloodstream their blood will become contaminated with the Hepatitis Virus.

As you can see Heroin is a very addictive and dangerous drug that can lead to you doing a lot of dangerous things to get your next hit of Heroin. That is why you should never use Heroin to get high.

My beautiful female; listed below are some of the other names used for Heroin.

- Birdie Powder
- Black Tar
- Ferry Dust
- Black Pearl
- H
- Brown Sugar
- HRN
- Hell Dust
- Joy Flakes
- Number 4
- Number 8
- Smack
- Red Chicken

- Mexican Mud
- Moon Rock
- Brick Gum
- Aunt Hazel
- Red Eagle
- Hard Candy
- Mexican Horse
- H Caps
- White Boy
- Mud
- Brown Crystal
- Chinese Red
- Tar
- Blow
- Hope Dope
- Trash
- White Nurse
- Salt
- White Junk
- Boy
- Charlie
- Dog Food
- Hairy
- Junk
- Life Saver
- Golden Girl
- The Beast
- Noise
- Hero
- The Witch
- Big Harry
- Hell Dust
- H- Bomb
- Raw Hide
- Hot Dope
- Reindeer Dust

- Flea Powder
- Bombita
- Mexican Brown
- Nod
- Dirt
- Mortal Combat
- TNT
- Spider
- Bull Dog
- Heroina
- P-Funk
- White Horse
- Tigre Blanco
- Primo

Also, if a person was to mix Heroin with other drugs that combination will have its own name too. Listed below are some of those combinations and their names.

- "Belushi" is Heroin and Cocaine
- "Chasing The Dragon" is Heroin and Crack Cocaine
- "China White" is Heroin and Fentanyl
- "Dynamite" is Heroin and Cocaine
- "Eight Ball" is Heroin and Crack Cocaine
- "Goofball" is Heroin and Cocaine
- "New Jack Swing" is Heroin and Morphine
- "Cotton Brothers" is Heroin, Cocaine, and Morphine
- "Flamethrower" is Heroin, Cocaine, and Tobacco
- "Murder One" is Heroin and Cocaine
- "TNT" is Heroin and Fentanyl
- "Smoking Gun" is Heroin and Cocaine
- "He – She" is Heroin and Cocaine
- "Magic" is Heroin and Fentanyl
- "The Bomb" is Heroin and Fentanyl
- "Five Way" is Heroin, Cocaine, Methamphetamine, Rohypnol, and Alcohol

My beautiful female you should know that if anyone was to take any of the combinations listed above that person will experience side effects from each and every drugs in that combination.

Remember, your body is a rare and precious jewel and a rare and precious jewel should be cherished and protected from harm and danger at all times by you. Using Heroin to get high is not an act of cherishing and protecting your rare and precious jewel.

MARIJUANA

My beautiful female you will meet a lot of people who will stress that Marijuana is safe. Some people will even say that Marijuana has no negative side effects unlike other illegal drugs people use. You will even meet people who will say they have smoked Marijuana for years and even decades and they are just fine.

The reason why they say that is because they cannot see what is going on in the inside of their body. For those of you who do not know what Marijuana is let me explain to you what it is. Marijuana is the flower bud of the Cannabis Sativa Plant.

This plant has several different chemicals in it. The chemical that gives user that euphoric feeling is *Delta-9- Tetrahydrocannabinol* (THC). Each strain of Marijuana contains a different level of THC as well as a different sensation. Sometimes the different strains of Marijuana are cross bred to create a new strain of Marijuana.

When a person smokes Marijuana that person causes the chemical THC to enter into their body through their lungs. Once THC is in their bloodstream it will work its way through their body.

My beautiful female some of the short term side effects a person can experience from using Marijuana to get high are:

- Loss of short term memory
- Learning disability
- Distorted perception of vision
- Distorted perception of time
- Irregular period
- Increased heart rate
- Loss of coordination

- Blood shot eyes
- Hunger (Munchies)
- Dry mouth
- Anxiety
- Paranoia
- Fear
- Decrease levels of testosterone in males
- Lack of coordination
- Slow reaction
- Addiction
- Hallucination
- Lack of concentration
- Increase levels of testosterone in females

Some of the long term side effects a person can experience from smoking Marijuana to get high is:

- Depression (some of these individuals already suffers from a mild form of depression)
- Schizophrenia (some of these individuals already suffers from a mild form of mental illness)
- Lack of muscle control
- Lack of judgment
- Impaired driving skills
- Psychological dependence
- Difficulty listening effectively
- Intense anxiety attacks
- Lesion on the brain
- Mood swings
- Impaired immune system
- Intense panic attacks
- Deteriorating lungs
- Breathing problems
- Lung infection
- Increase in blood pressure

My precious female if you choose to smoke Marijuana you will damage the air sacs on your lung. Once the air sacs are damaged from smoking Marijuana oxygen is unable to be transported into your bloodstream like it should be. This will cause your heart to have to work harder.

Another thing that can happen because you chose to smoke Marijuana to get high is that your athletic performance will not be at its best. All because your body will not be able to take in the required amount of oxygen it needs. This is happening because your air sacs are damaged from the Marijuana you have smoked. Plus, your body will take longer to heal from injuries.

A third thing that can happen is you can cause damage to your developing brain. Once the brain cells are damaged they are damaged for life. That is why it is not a very good idea for a tweens or teen girls and boys to smoke Marijuana. If you are a tween or a teen your brain is still developing which means you are damaging the undeveloped brain cells that you currently have. Just so you know a brain is not fully developed until you have reached twenty-five years of age.

My beautiful female you can also develop respiratory problems from smoking Marijuana. Some of the respiratory problems you can develop are:
- Lung cancer
- Chest pain
- Mucus builds up

You should also know that smoking Marijuana can cause changes in your physical appearance. Listed below are some of the physical changes you can experience from smoking Marijuana.
- You can gain weight from over eating because you have the munchies (the desire to eat).
- Your skin loses its natural glow.
- The whites of your eyes become dull in color.
- Your finger nails become discolored.
- Your lips become discolored.

My beautiful female listed below are some of the different strains of Marijuana.
- Bahia Black Head
- Apollo Mist

- Thunder Fuckin Wonder
- Super Silver Spice
- Super Kush
- White Widow
- Voodoo
- Ultra Skunk
- Twisted Fruit
- Sugar Babe
- Sour Wonder
- Blueberry Blast
- Island Sweet Skunk
- Gypsy Kiss
- Hawaiian Sativa
- Heavy Duty Fruity
- G13 Blue Widow
- Lemon Skunk
- Master Kush
- Lion heart
- Love Potion #1
- King's Kross
- KGB
- Jamaican Pearl
- Double Dutch Haze Skunk
- Blue Velvet
- Cherry Bomb
- Blue Skunk
- Early Brambleberry
- Early Misty
- Grapefruit Haze
- Grapeskunk
- Hoosier Hoot'n'Hollar
- Mongolian Indica
- Neon Skunk
- Northern Lights #1
- Northern Lights #9
- Rock Star

- Reeferman's Space Queen
- Purple Thai
- Cinderella 88
- Ultimate Peak
- Tropical Timewrap
- Tanzanian Magic
- Sunshine Daydream
- Orange Peako Cambodian
- Mr Bubble
- New Purple Power
- Mindfuck
- Ice Princess
- Bubblejuice
- Blue God
- Apple Pie

My beautiful female these are just a few of the many different strains of Marijuana that are available. Just so you know Marijuana can be a depressant or a stimulant depending on the type of Marijuana you have.

My precious female just because Marijuana does not attack your body extremely fast or very aggressively does not mean it is not attacking your body. For those individuals who use flavored blunt wrappers you are causing even more harm and damage to your body because of the chemicals used on the blunt wrappers. Which means not only will the person have to deal with the side effects from the Marijuana they will have to deal with the side effects from the chemical used on the blunt wrapper.

Listed below are some of the other names used for Marijuana.

- African Bush
- Flower Top
- Weed
- Roots
- Pot
- Mary Jane
- Kushempeng
- Chicago Green

- Broccoli
- Ashes
- Aunt Mary
- Doja
- Shiva
- Grass
- Texas Tea
- Herb
- Hooch
- Indian Hay
- Dro
- Wheat
- Roach
- Dagga
- J
- Kush
- Pine
- Dobie
- Hay
- Supergrass
- Dew
- Root
- Reefer
- Hash
- Homegrown
- Love Leaf
- Indian Hemp
- Trees

Also, if a person was to mix Marijuana with other drugs that combination will have its own name too. Listed below are some of those combinations and their names.
- "Woolie Blunt" is Marijuana and Crack Cocaine
- "Cocoa Puff" is Marijuana and Cocaine
- "El Diablo" is Marijuana, Cocaine, and Heroin
- "Squirrel" is Marijuana, Cocaine, and PCP
- "TIO" is Marijuana, and Cocaine

- "El Diablito" is Marijuana, Cocaine, Heroin, and PCP
- "Greek Joint" is Marijuana cigarette and Cocaine
- "51" is Marijuana and Crack Cocaine
- "A-Bomb" is Marijuana and Heroin
- "Candy Sticks" is Marijuana and Cocaine powder
- "P-Dog" is Marijuana and Cocaine
- "Sherman Sticks" is Marijuana and Crack Cocaine
- "Bazooka" is Marijuana and Cocaine
- "Caviar" is Marijuana and Cocaine

My beautiful female if anyone was to use any of the combinations listed above they will experience side effects from each of the drugs in that combination.

Remember, your body is a rare and precious jewel and a rare and precious jewel should be cherished and protected from harm and danger by you at all times. Using Marijuana to get high is not an act of cherishing and protection your rare and precious jewel from harm and danger.

CRACK COCAINE

My beautiful female Crack Cocaine is a very addictive drug that can cause your rare and precious jewel a lot of harm and damage. Crack Cocaine gets its name from the cracking sound it makes when you smoke it.

When a person smoke Crack Cocaine to get high it will cause him or her to experience several different negative side effects. Some of the side effects a person can experience from using Crack Cocaine to get high are:
- Increase in blood pressure
- Increase in heart rate
- Nausea
- Vomiting
- Anxiety
- Convulsions
- Respiratory problems
- Depression
- Craving Crack Cocaine
- Muscle spasm
- Paranoia
- Mood swings
- Seizures
- Loss of appetite
- Damage to your lungs
- Damage to your nasal septum
- Weight loss
- Swelling of the mucus membrane
- Bleeding of the mucus membrane
- Damage to the nasal cavity

Some of the long term side effects a person can experience from using Crack Cocaine to get high are:
- Extreme weight loss
- Death
- Paranoia
- Being delusional
- Impaired judgment
- Lung trauma
- Constricted blood vessels
- Cardiac arrest
- Insomnia
- Heart Damage
- Liver Damage
- Kidney Damage
- Seizures
- Bleeding of your lungs
- Tooth decay
- Malnutrition
- Damage to the nasal cavity

Also, when the high from the Crack Cocaine has worn off some abuser of Crack Cocaine will begin to feel depressed. Now that the individual feels depressed they will want to smoke more Crack Cocaine so they can feel that euphoric feeling again instead of the depressed feeling they feel. As you can see this will become a vicious cycle. The desire to make the depress feeling go away will lead to that individual using more and more Crack Cocaine.

Now that the Crack Cocaine Addict is increasing the amount of Crack Cocaine he or she uses it will cause that person to spend more and more money to support their Crack Cocaine addiction. Now that the individual is using more and more Crack Cocaine their chances of overdosing on this drug is greater.

My beautiful female; when a Crack Cocaine Addict decides to stop using Crack Cocaine he or she will experience withdrawal symptoms. For those of you who do not know what withdrawal symptoms are let me explain it to you. Withdrawal symptoms

are the different physical and psychological changes the body will go through when a person stop using Crack Cocaine (or other drugs) to get high. Listed below are some of the withdrawal symptoms a person can experience when he or she stop using Crack Cocaine.
- Fatigue
- Depression
- Lack of motivation
- Muscle pain
- Insomnia
- Disturbing Visions
- Hallucinations
- Mood swings
- Craving Crack Cocaine
- Agitation
- Irritability
- Anxiety
- Violent outbursts
- Nausea
- Vomiting
- Uncontrollable shaking
These are just a few of the withdrawal symptoms a Crack Cocaine Addict can experience once he or she stops using Crack Cocaine to get high. Also, the length of time the individual will experience withdrawal symptoms will varies among each individual.
My beautiful female if a female chooses to use Crack Cocaine while she is pregnant she can experience several undesirable things such as:
- Premature labor
- Premature delivery
- Still birth (your baby being born dead)
- Miscarriages
If she continues to use Crack Cocaine during her full pregnancy her baby can suffer from:
- Cerebral Palsy

- Learning disability
- Stroke
- Seizures
- Mental retardation
- Autism
- Hearing impaired
- Vision impaired

My beautiful female; listed below are some of the other names used for Crack Cocaine.
- B.J's.
- Crack
- Beemers
- Chewies
- Devil Dandruff
- Boulders
- Bones
- Casper The Ghost
- Crunch And Munch
- Hail
- Love
- Schoolcraft
- Top Gun
- Stones
- Hot Cakes
- Nuggets
- Rock Star
- Jelly Beans
- Garbage Rocks
- Eyeball Poppers
- Crack Coolers (crack soaked in wine coolers)
- Chocolate Ecstasy (crack turned brown because of the chocolate milk mix used in the cooking process)
- Bolo
- Bings
- White Ball
- Ice Cubes

- Sleet
- Rock Attack
- Troop
- Gravel
- Rocks Of Hell
- Roosters
- The Devil
- White Ghost
- Cookies
- Rox

Also, if someone was to mix Crack Cocaine with other drugs that combination will have its own name too. Listed below are some of those combinations and their names.

- "Chocolate Rock" is Crack Cocaine and Heroin
- "Whack" is Crack Cocaine and PCP
- "51" is Crack Cocaine and Marijuana
- "Tar" is Crack Cocaine and Heroin
- "Chasing The Dragon" is Crack Cocaine and Heroin
- "Mexican Speedball" is Crack Cocaine and Methamphetamine
- "Sherman Sticks" is Crack Cocaine and Marijuana
- "Cocktail" is Crack Cocaine and Marijuana
- "Eight Ball" is Crack Cocaine and Heroin
- "Sheet Rocking" is Crack Cocaine and LSD

My beautiful female you should know that if anyone was to use one of these combinations that person will experience side effects from each drug in that combination.

Remember, your body is a rare and precious jewel and a rare and precious jewel should be cherished and protected from harm and danger by you at all time. Using Crack Cocaine to get high is not an act of cherishing and protecting your rare and precious jewel from harm and danger.

LSD

(Lysergic Acid Diethylamide)

Lysergic Acid Diethylamide also known as LSD is a synthetic hallucinogenic drug. LSD is a colorless and odorless drug that has a slight bitter taste. This drug is usually sold as a liquid, laced blotter paper, laced sugar cubes, laced gelatin squares, or table. My beautiful female LSD is an unpredictable drug. This drug has caused people to do things that were very illogical. Sometime their actions have led to their death. The severity of the side effects a person will experience will depend on several things such as:

- The amount of LSD the person has taken
- Their personality
- Their mental state
- The environment the individual was in when he or she took the drug

Some of the short term side effects a person can experience from using LSD to get high are:

- Dizziness
- Feeling different emotions at the same time
- Increased heart rate
- Increased blood pressure
- Tremors
- Sweating
- Loss of appetite
- Insomnia
- Hallucination
- Dry mouth

- Rapid mood swings

If a large dose of LSD is taken the individual will experience:

- Becoming delusional
- Hallucinations
- The belief of hearing colors
- The belief of seeing sounds
- Panic
- Fear
- Paranoia

Some of the long term side effects a person can experience from using a high dosage LSD to get high are:

- Flashbacks
- Clinical depression
- Schizophrenia

When using LSD the individual will experience what is known as "Tripping". When "Tripping" you will experience:

- Being anxious
- Colors are extremely vivid
- Everything seems to be moving in slow motion
- Extreme mental changes (mood swings)
- Paranoia

Another form of "Tripping" the individual will experience is a bad "Tripping" experience. A bad "Tripping" experience has been described as "A Living Nightmare" and "A Living Hell". The only way to get out of a bad "Tripping" experience is for the high from the LSD to wear off. Just so you know the high from LSD can last for hours. Which means the person will have to endure the horrors of that bad "Tripping" experience for however many hours your high last. If you are wondering is there anything a person can do to speed up the process? The answer is absolutely not. That person will have to endure the horrors of that bad "Tripping" experience.

You should know that you will never know what "Tripping" experience you are going to have until you have it.

My beautiful female; there have been people who have jumped out of a window while "Tripping" on LSD. Also, some people

have become physically violent towards themselves and other people around them while "Tripping" on LSD.
Listed below are some of the other names used for LSD.
- Angles In The Sky
- Acid
- Blue Acid
- Blue Moon
- Black Sunshine
- Cupcakes
- Dots
- Kool Aide
- Blue Mist
- Golden Dragon
- Lime Acid
- Haze
- Heavenly Blue
- L
- Orange Haze
- Mind Detergent
- Pink Panther
- Sunshine
- Yellow Sunshine
- Purple Haze
- Royal Blues
- Strawberry Fields
- Pink Robot
- Hawk
- Brown Bomber
- Blotter
- Black Star
- Bart Simpson
- Angel Tears
- Alice
- Beast
- Blotter Cubes
- Blue Fly

- Chinese Dragon
- Coffee
- Electric
- Blue Heaven
- Hats
- Mighty Quinn
- Orange Wedge
- Pink Blotter
- Purple Love
- Zen
- Paper Acid
- Peace Tablets
- Optical Illusion
- Sugar Cubes
- White Lightning
- Wedding Bells
- Gods Flesh
- Blue Microdot
- Electric Kool Aid
- South Park
- Sugar Lumps

Also, if an individual was to mix LSD with other drugs that combination will have its own name too. Listed below are some of those combinations and their names.

- "Troll" is LSD and Ecstasy
- "Rocket Fuel" is LSD and Cocaine
- "Frisco Speedball" is LSD (small amount), Cocaine, and Heroin
- "Black Acid" is LSD and PCP
- "Candy Flippin On A String" is LSD, Ecstasy, and Cocaine
- "Candy Flipping" is LSD and Ecstasy
- "Sheet Rocking" is LSD and Crack Cocaine

My precious female if anyone was to take any of the combinations listed above that person will experience side effects from each drug in that combination.

Remember, your body is a rare and precious jewel and a rare and precious jewel should be cherished and protected from harm and danger by you at all times. Using LSD to get high will cause harm and damage to your rare and precious jewel.

GHB
(Gamma Hydroxy Butyrate)

Gamma Hydroxy Butyrate (GHB) also known as *The Date Rape Drug* is being used for recreational use. My beautiful female you should know that taking GHB for recreational use can be very dangerous. Your body will absorb this drug in approximately 15 minutes after taking it. Plus, it will cause the individual to be uninhibited when it comes to doing thing that person will normally not do. GHB will cause people to act before thinking; which can lead to people experiencing some undesirable circumstances.

Using GHB to get high can have negative side effects on the body. Some of the short term side effects a person can experience from taking GHB to get high are:

- Lightheadedness
- Dangerously decreased heart rate
- Vomiting
- Hallucinations
- Dizziness
- Nausea
- Headaches
- Drowsiness
- Weakness
- Agitation

Taking GHB with alcohol can be extremely dangerous. Sometime it can even be deadly. Some of the side effects a person can experience from taking GHB with alcohol are:

- Death

- Coma
- Mental confusion
- Breathing difficulties
- Slurred speech

A person can also overdose on GHB when mixed with alcohol. My beautiful female you can also die if you take GHB in high dosages.

I want you to know by taking GHB to get high you have just made yourself an easy target for:

- Sexual assault
- Rape
- Robbery
- Murder

These things can take place because of the mental state you will be in because of the GHB you had taken. This is why you should not use GHB to get high.

My lovely female; there are some people who use GHB as a Date Rape Drug. These individuals choose to use this drug because it can cause the person they drugged to become incoherent to what is going on around them and to them. It can also cause that individual to pass out. Plus, the person who is drugged with GHB can easily be persuaded to do things they may not normally do or want to do.

You should know that all drinks can be spiked with GHB; soda, juice, water, milk, alcohol or any other drink you may have. If you are wondering can they spike food with GHB; the answer is yes.

Listed below are some of the other names used for GHB.

- G
- Liquid Ecstasy
- Georgia Home Boy
- Grievous Bodily Harm
- Scoop
- Water
- Fantasy
- Erotica

- Heaven
- Salty Water
- Easy Lay
- Sleep 500
- G- Riffic
- Beauty
- Bedtime
- Everclear
- Liquid X
- Zoom
- Great Hormones At Bedtime
- Sleep
- Organic Quaalude

My beautiful female just so you now GHB is made from *Gamma Butyrolacetone* (GBL). When GBL is ingested the body will convert it into GHB. Listed below are some of the other names used for GBL.

- Blue Nitro
- Thunder Nectar
- Revivarant
- RenewTrient
- Revitalize Plus
- Invigorate
- Firewater

Also, if a person mix GHB with other drugs that combination has its own name too. Listed below are some of the combinations and their names.

- "Max" is GHB and Amphetamine
- "Everclear" is GHB and Cocaine
- "Soap" is GHB, Cocaine, and Methamphetamine
- "Water" is GHB, Marijuana, PCP, and Methamphetamine

If someone was to take any of the combinations listed above that person will experience side effects from each of the drugs in that combination.

My beautiful female your body is a rare and precious jewel and a rare and precious jewel should be cherished and protected from

Lora McDuffie

harm and danger. Using GHB to get high is not an act of cherishing or protecting your rare and precious jewel.

ROHYPNOL

Rohypnol is also known as the *Date Rape Drug* and *Flunitrazepam*. This is a very powerful sedative that is prescribed as a sleeping pill. This drug will give you a sleepy and drunk feeling at the same time that can last up to 8 hours. It has been known to last longer than 8 hours in some people.

My beautiful female some of the side effects a person can experience from using Rohypnol to get high are:

- Nightmares
- Tremors
- Drowsiness
- Confusion
- Headaches
- Dizziness
- Memory loss
- Aggression
- Easily excited
- Impaired judgment
- Impaired motor skills
- Blackouts
- Memory loss

Taking Rohypnol with alcohol is a very dangerous thing to do. Not only is it dangerous it can also be deadly. Some of the side effects a person can experience from take Rohypnol with Alcohol are:

- Death
- Decrease in blood pressure
- Hallucinations
- Gastrointestinal disturbances

- Frequent urination
- Memory loss
- Blackouts
- Impaired motor skills

Once a person stops using Rohypnol to get high that individual will experience withdrawal symptoms. Listed below are some of the withdrawal symptoms a person can experience when he or she stops using Rohypnol to get high.

- Headaches
- Convulsions
- Seizures
- Hallucination
- Muscle pain
- Confusion

These are just a few of the withdrawal symptoms a person can experience once he or she stops using Rohypnol to get high. Also, the length of time a person will experience withdrawal symptoms will vary between each individual.

I want you to know that some people will use Rohypnol as a Date Rape Drug. This drug is being used because it impairs the person's motor skills and it causes blackouts. In some cases people have experienced memory loss with blackouts. These are just a few reasons why people use this drug as a date rape drug.

Just so you know some of the Rohypnol caplets that are being used to spike female's drinks will turn their drink blue. If you are drinking a dark colored drink you will not notice the color change. With that being said; you should never drink a drink you have left unattended. Nor should you drink a drink that a waiter or a waitress did not bring you. Also, you should not drink a drink that you did not see the person fix. If your drink was spiked with Rohypnol the person who spiked your drink can rape you, rob you, abduct you, or murder you. Or the person who spiked your drink can do all four things to you. I want you to know that any drink you drink can be spiked with Rohypnol; soda, juice, water, alcohol or any other drink you may have. If you are wondering can someone spike your food with Rohypnol the answer is yes?

My beautiful female; listed below are some of the other names used for Rohypnol.

- Rope
- Roach 2
- Getting Roached
- Circles
- Mexican Valium
- Forget Me Pill
- Ruffies
- Rophy
- Lunch Money Drug
- Date Rape Drug
- Rib
- Roofenol
- R-2
- La Rocha
- Row- Shay
- Circles
- Reynolds
- Roofies
- Ruffles
- Wolfies
- Forget Me Drug
- Robutal

Also, if someone was to mix Rohypnol with other drugs that combination will have its own name too. Listed below are some of the combinations and their names.

- "Five Way" is Rohypnol, Cocaine, Heroin, Methamphetamine, and Alcohol
- "Rib" is Rohypnol and Ecstasy
- "Rope" is Rohypnol and Marijuana

My precious female you should know if you were to take any of the combinations listed above you will experience side effects from each of the drugs in that combination.

Lora McDuffie

Remember, your body is a rare and precious jewel and a rare and precious jewel should be cherished and protected from harm and danger by you at all times. Using Rohypnol to get high is not act of cherishing and protecting your rare and precious jewel.

PCP

(Phenylcyclohexyl Piperidine)

Phenylcyclohexyl Piperidine, also known as PCP; was created to be used as an intravenous anesthetic. Its use was discontinued because of the very negative side effects the patient would experience out way the positive use of the drug. In some case the patient will experience the negative side effects days, weeks, and even months after they have been treated with PCP. Also, some patients became suicidal after being treated with PCP.

PCP is a drug that has a distinct bitter taste. It can be snorted, intravenously injected into the veins, smoked, or taken orally.

Some of the side effects a person can experience when taking a small dosage of PCP are:

- Numbness of the legs
- Numbness of the arms
- Feeling detached from your surroundings
- Shallow breathing
- Slurred speech
- Profuse sweating
- Lack of coordination
- Blood shot eyes
- Staggering

Some of the side effects a person can experience when taking a moderate amount of PCP to get high are:

- A blank stare
- Rapid eye movement
- Involuntary eye movement
- Exaggerated gait foot movement (trotting like a hoarse)

- Irritability
- Sever mood swings
- Anxiety
- Feeling of upcoming doom
- Disoriented
- Paranoia
- Confusion
- Restlessness
- Violence
- Hostility
- Behavior resembling schizophrenia
- Mental disturbance

List below are some of the side effects a person can experience from taking a large dose of PCP to get high are:
- Coma
- Death
- Seizures
- Decrease in blood pressure
- Decrease in pulse rate
- Difficulty with inhaling and exhaling
- Hallucinations
- Convulsion
- Being delusional
- Behavior resembling schizophrenia
- Mental torment
- Vomiting
- Nausea
- Blurred vision
- Distorted perception of sounds
- Distorted perception of vision

My beautiful female using PCP can cause problems with your growth and development because of the negative effects it will have on your hormones; which can lead to deformities in some people.

If a person was to use PCP for a long period of time he or she can experience:

- Weight loss
- Memory loss
- Depression

Also, some people who are high on PCP and in a controlled setting or detained in a hospital can become very violent towards themselves as well as others. As you can see taking PCP can be very dangerous to you physically and mentally. Plus, it may cause you to become a danger to other people.

My beautiful female some of the other names used for PCP are listed below.

- Angel Dust
- Butt Naked
- Detroit Pink
- Magic Dust
- Cliff Hanger
- Cadillac
- Dummy Dust
- Green Tea
- Heaven and Hell
- Lethal Weapon
- Lemon 714
- Mad Dog
- Lovely
- Monkey Dust
- Orange Crystal
- Peace Pill
- Pig Killer
- Tic Tac
- TT1
- TT2
- TT3
- Yellow Flower
- Wolf
- Rocket Fuel
- STP
- Peter Pan

- Purple Rain
- Mean Green
- Little Ones
- K-Blast
- Juice
- KJ
- Energizer
- Goon Dust
- Elephant Tranquilizer
- Cyclone
- Busy Bee
- Angel
- Angel Hair
- Amoeba
- Animal Tranq
- Gorilla Tab
- Horse Tranquilizer
- Kools
- T-Buzz
- Super Kool

Also, if a person was to mix PCP with other drugs those combinations will have their own name too. Listed below are some of those combinations and their names.

- "Elephant Flipping" is PCP and Ecstasy
- "Jet Fuel" is PCP and Methamphetamine
- "Jim Jones" is PCP, Cocaine, and Marijuana
- "Black Acid" is PCP and LSD
- "LBJ" is PCP, LSD, and Heroin
- "Poro" is PCP and Heroin
- "Space Ball" is PCP and Cocaine
- "Squirrel" is PCP, Cocaine, and Marijuana
- "Wicky" is PCP, Cocaine, and Marijuana
- "El Diablito" is PCP, Cocaine, Marijuana, and Heroin
- "Domex" is PCP and Ecstasy

My beautiful female if someone was to take any of these combinations that person will experience side effects from each of the drugs in that combination.

Remember, your body is a rare and precious jewel and a rare and precious jewel should be cherished and protected from harm and danger at all times by you. When you use PCP to get high you will cause harm and damage to your rare and precious jewel.

COCAINE

Cocaine is a drug that comes from the leaf of the Erythroxylon Coca Bush. This is a drug that affects the Central Nervous System. The Central Nervous System (CNS) is the part of the brain that controls movement, emotions, and behavioral changes.

My beautiful female Cocaine is a highly addictive and a very dangerous drug. When taking Cocaine to get high you can cause damage to different parts of your body. The parts of the body that you can damage are:

- The brain
- The heart
- The respiratory system

The way Cocaine affects the body is determined by several different things such as:

- The amount of Cocaine taken
- The purity of the drug
- Was the drug taken with alcohol?
- Was the drug taken with other drugs?
- The individual weight
- The individual height
- The individual mental state

When Cocaine has reached the brain it causes a chemical imbalance in the brain. The chemical in the brain that is affected by Cocaine is *Dopamine*. Dopamine regulates movement, emotions, learning, and pleasure.

When a person uses Cocaine to get high they have just increased their chances of having a heart attack. The reason why that individual is able to have a massive heart attack is because Cocaine stops the flow of oxygen in the blood. That lack of oxygen will restricts the flow of blood that goes to your heart. If the heart is unable to receive oxygenized blood it will stop beating. Also, when you use Cocaine it will weaken your arterial walls and cause your blood vessels to become constricted. Having your blood vessels constricted can lead to you having a heart attack. If Cocaine is being inhaled directly into the respiratory system you will develop Chronic Bronchitis. In addition to having respiratory problems you will have excessive coughing. Sometimes you will even develop chest pains. Plus, you will accumulate a lot of mucus in your chest and throat.

My beautiful female you must know that a person can overdose on Cocaine. For those of you who do not know what it means to overdose on Cocaine (or other drugs) let me explain it to you. When a person overdose on Cocaine that person has taken an amount of Cocaine that their heart is unable to handle. Because their heart is unable to handle the drugs he or she had taken it will stop beating. In some cases their heart will explode in their chest cavity. Once their heart has stopped beating or exploded in their chest cavity he or she will die.

Sometimes the person who is overdosing on Cocaine can receive medical attention and it can save their life. In some cases the person can receive medical attention and the person still dies.

Some of the negative side effects a person can experience from using Cocaine to get high are:

- Unusual muscle weakness
- Tremors
- Vomiting
- Headaches
- Nausea
- Tingling in the hands
- Tingling in the feet
- Numbness in the arms
- Numbness in the legs
- Stomach pain
- Fainting

- Tooth decay
- Lightheadedness
- Dilated Pupils
- Difficulty urinated
- Irritability
- Irregular heart beat
- Nervousness
- Easily excited
- Agitation
- Mood swings
- Metal disturbances
- Excessive coughing
- Excessive mucus buildup

If a person was to use large quantities of Cocaine to get high he or she can experience some of the negative side effects listed below.
- Death
- Coma
- Kidney disease
- Liver disease
- Stroke
- Autoimmune Disease
- Overdose
- Constricted blood vessels
- Chronic Bronchitis
- High blood pressure
- Massive heart attack
- Weaken heart arterial walls

My precious female when a person decides to stop using Cocaine that person will experience withdrawal symptoms. Listed below are some of the withdrawal symptoms a person can experience.
- Depression
- Fatigue
- Irritability
- Vivid dreams

- Restlessness
- Sluggishness
- Easily agitated
- Suicidal thoughts
- Confusion
- Blurred vision
- Chills
- Lack of focus
- Increase appetite
- Weight gain
- Achy body
- Insomnia
- Tremors
- Craving Cocaine
- Muscle pain
- Mood swing
- Disturbing dreams
- Exhaustion
- Paranoia

These are just a few of the withdrawal symptoms you can experience once you stop using Cocaine to get high. If a female was to use Cocaine while she is pregnant she can cause her baby to be still born. For those of you who do not know what still born is; it is your baby being born dead. Another thing the baby can experience because the mom was using Cocaine while she was pregnant is physical deformities. Plus, the baby will become addicted to Cocaine just like their mother. Using Cocaine to get high while pregnant is very damaging for the baby physically and mentally. Plus, it can lead to the death of your baby.
Listed below are some of the other names used for Cocaine.

- Big C
- Big Rush
- Candy C
- Girlfriend
- Green Gold
- Happy Dust

- Nose Candy
- Scorpian
- Tar Dust
- Snow Bird
- White Girl
- Snow Cones
- Lady Snow
- Love Affair
- C Game
- C Dust
- Charlie
- Schoolboy
- Icing
- Carnie
- Nose Powder
- Snow White
- Bazooka
- Henry VIII
- Florida Snow
- Foo Dust
- Peruvian Flake
- California Cornflakes
- Happy Trails
- Happy Powder
- Nose Stuff
- Scottie
- Pimp
- Carrie

Also, if you were to mix Cocaine with other drugs those combinations will have their own name too. Listed below are some of the combinations and their names.
- "Murder One" is Cocaine and Heroin
- "Snowball" is Cocaine and Heroin
- "Snow Seal" is Cocaine and Amphetamine
- "Monkey" is Cocaine and Tobacco
- "Goofball" is Cocaine and Heroin

- "Belushi" is Cocaine and Heroin
- "Croak" is Cocaine and Methamphetamine
- "Frisco Speedball" is Cocaine, Heroin, and LSD (a small amount)
- "Smoking Gun" is Cocaine and Heroin
- "Squirrel" is Cocaine, PCP, and Marijuana
- "Flamethrowers" is Cocaine, Heroin, and Tobacco
- "Five Way" is Cocaine, Heroin, Methamphetamine, Rohypnol, and Alcohol
- "Dynamite" is Cocaine and Heroin
- "Pemos" is Cocaine and Marijuana
- "Wicky" is Cocaine, PCP, and Marijuana

My beautiful female if you were to take any of the combinations listed above you will experience side effects from each of the drugs in that combination.

Remember, your body is a rare and precious jewel and a rare and precious jewel should be cherished and protected from harm and danger. Using Cocaine to get high you will cause harm and damage to your rare and precious jewel.

DXM

(Dextromethorphan)

DXM (*Dextromethorphan*) is a synthetic form of codeine that is used as a cough suppressant in over the counter cough medicine. This drug affects the part of the brain that triggers the cough. Some people will take over the counter cough medicine to get high because they like the sedated affect it has on the body. The drug *Dextromethorphan,* also known as DXM; will give it abuser some of the same affects as drinking alcohol.

When taking DXM for recreational use (for fun) you will go through four different plateaus.

The First Plateau

1.5 – 2.5 mg/kg

This dosage is the weakest. Some of the side effects a person can experience from the first plateau are:

- Lightheadedness
- A little intoxicate

The Second Plateau

2.5 – 7.5 mg/kg

Some of the side effects a person can experience from the second plateau are:

- Difficulty talking
- Slurred Speech
- Difficulty focusing
- Short term memory is impaired
- Hallucination
- Impaired coordination
- Double vision

- Nausea
The Third Plateau
7.5 – 15 mg/kg
Some of the side effects a person can experience from the third plateau are:
- Impaired sensory input
- Delusional
- Disoriented
- Recall of suppressed memory
- Illogical thinking
- Harmful to oneself
- Hallucination
- Mental disturbance
- Confusion
The Fourth Plateau
15+ mg/kg
This is the strongest plateau. Some of the side effects a person can experience from the fourth plateau are:
- Death
- Brain damage
- Seizures
- Psychological problems
- Dissociation of the mind
- Dissociation of the body
- Physical problems
- Vomiting
- Irrational thinking
- Impaired contact with external senses
- Impaired judgment
- Loss of coordination
- Dizziness
My beautiful female when a person decides to stop using DXM to get high that person will experience withdrawal symptoms. Listed below are some of the withdrawal symptoms a person can experience when he or she stop using DXM to get high.
- Depression

- Anxiety
- Insomnia
- Vomiting
- Suicide thoughts
- Diarrhea
- Weight loss
- Restlessness
- Headaches
- Nightmares
- Upset stomach

These are just a few of the withdrawal symptom a person can experience once he or she stops using DXM to get high. As you can see using DXM can be very dangerous and even deadly.

My beautiful female; listed below are some of the other names used for DXM.

- Skittles
- Triple C
- Tussin
- Bromage
- Dex
- Robo
- Red Devil
- Tex M
- D
- Brome

Remember, your body is a rare and precious jewel and a rare and precious jewel should be cherished and protected from harm and danger by you at all times. By using DXM to get high you will cause harm and damage to your rare and precious jewel.

CRYSTAL METH
(*Crystal Methamphetamine Hydrochloride*)

Crystal Meth (*Crystal Methamphetamine Hydrochloride*) is a psychoactive stimulant drug that is highly addictive. Crystal Meth causes the Central Nervous System to release large amounts of the chemical in the brain called *Dopamine*. Dopamine regulates mood, body movement, learning, and pleasure.

Crystal Meth is a clear chunk of *Methamphetamine* that is snorted, smoked, or injected into the bloodstream. The high that you can get from Crystal Meth can last up to eight hours, but it has been known to last longer in some people.

My beautiful female using Crystal Meth can cause your body a lot of damage. Some of the immediate side effects a person can experience from using Crystal Meth to get high are:

- Irritability
- Nervousness
- Panic attacks
- Hostility
- Dry skin
- Hallucinations
- Insomnia
- Violent behavior
- Seizures
- Erratic behavior
- Convulsions
- Paranoia
- Loss of appetite
- Increase heart rate

- Increase in body temperature
- Increase in blood pressure
- Tremors
- Dry mouth
- Cramps
- Tooth decay
- Rapid weight loss
- Suicidal tendencies
- Sunken face
- Itchy skin
- Nausea
- Sores
- Illogical thinking
- Mood swings
- Confusion
- Blurred vision
- Sever headaches
- Blemished skin
- Dizziness
- Irregular heart beat
- Excessive sweating

Some of the long term side effects a person can experience from using Crystal Meth to get high are:
- Damage to your brain
- Damage to your liver
- Damage to the blood vessel of the heart
- Damage to your kidneys
- Damage to your lungs
- Damage to the tissue in the nasal cavity (this occurs from snorting Crystal Meth)
- High blood pressure
- Heart attacks
- Psychological dependency
- Exhaustion
- Heart failure
- Collapsed veins (this occurs from injecting Crystal Meth into

your veins)
- Damage to the lining of the nose (this occurs from snorting Crystal Meth)
- Damage to the lungs (this occurs from smoking Crystal Meth)
- Scarring of the body
- Malnutrition
- Anorexia
- Sores on skin
- Insomnia
- Kidney failure
- Low immune system
- Depression
- Anxiety
- Loss of memory
- Damage to your teeth
- Itchy skin
- Diarrhea
- Psychosis
- Stroke
- Jaw clenching
- Confusion
- Violent behavior

My precious female you should know that using Crystal Meth will literally age you. The longer you use Crystal Meth the older you will look. You will not look pretty during this premature aging process. You will look old and sickly.

Another thing you can experience from using Crystal Meth to get high is losing your teeth prematurely. This is known as *"Meth Mouth"*. If this was to happen to you there is one of two things you can do.

1st Thing You Can Do
Buy yourself some dentures and wear fake teeth for the rest of your life.

2nd Thing You Can Do
Spend the rest of your life with no teeth in your mouth.

Also, Crystal Meth will literally eat away brain tissue and leave holes in your brain.

My beautiful female I want you to know that going on a Crystal Meth binge is a very dangerous thing to do. For those of you who do not know what a Crystal Meth binge is let me explain it to you. When a person goes on a Crystal Meth binge this person will continuously and uncontrollably use Crystal Meth for days and even weeks. This person will use so much Crystal Meth to the point that the Crystal Meth will no longer produce the high he or she is striving for. The more Crystal Meth that person uses during the binge the less intense the high will be. Eventually; that person will no longer be able to get high from the Crystal Meth he or she is using.

After finishing a Crystal Meth binge that person will experience what is known as "Tweaking". For those of you who do not know what "Tweaking" is let me explain it to you. When "Tweaking" the individual will become psychotic or display psychotic behavior. He or she will experience horrific visions that appear to be real. This individual will be disconnected from reality. Also, some of the individuals will believe that bugs are crawling on them and crawling under their skin because of the intense itching he or she is having. There have been cases where some of these individuals have dug holes in their skin to try to get the bugs out (that do not exist). To make matter worst all of this is happening to the person while he or she is experiencing days and sometimes weeks of insomnia. As you can see using Crystal Meth damages you physically and mentally.

My beautiful female; when a person decides to stop using Crystal Meth to get high, he or she will have withdrawal symptoms. Listed below are some of the withdrawal symptoms a person can experience from using Crystal Meth.

- Anxiety
- Horrific dreams
- Exhaustion
- Fatigue
- Hunger
- Paranoia

- Irritability
- Mental confusion
- Depression
- Restlessness
- Agitation
- Insomnia
- Intense drug craving

These are just a few of the withdrawal symptoms a person can experience once he or she stops using Crystal Meth to get high.

My beautiful female I want you to know that a person can overdose on Crystal Meth. For those of you who do not know what overdosing is let me explain it to you. When a person overdose on Crystal Meth (or other drugs) that person has taken an amount that their heart is unable to handle. Because their heart is unable to handle the Crystal Meth he or she has taken it will stop beating. Once their heart has stopped beating he or she will die.

Listed below are some of the other names used for Crystal Meth.

- Chalk
- Crank
- Tina
- Glass
- D-Meth
- Shabu
- Crystal
- Batu
- Speed
- Ice
- Meth
- L.A. Glass
- Water
- Crystal Glass
- Quartz
- Blade
- Cristy
- Stove Top

- Shards
- Ventana
- Hot Ice
- Croak
- Crypto
- Super Ice

Also, if a person was to mix Crystal Meth with other drugs that combination will have its own name too. Listed below are some of the combinations and their names.

- "Chalk" is Crystal Meth, Cocaine, and Amphetamines
- "Bikers Coffee" is Crystal Meth and Coffee
- "Ice" is Crystal Meth, Cocaine, and Crack Cocaine
- "Meth Speedball" is Crystal Meth and Heroin
- "Mexican Speedball" is Crystal Meth and Crack Cocaine

My precious female if you take any of the combinations listed above you will experience side effects from each and every drug in that combination.

Remember, your body is a rare and precious jewel and a rare and precious jewel should be cherished and protected from harm and danger by you at all times. By using Crystal Meth to get high you will cause harm and damage to your rare and precious jewel.

ALCOHOL

My beautiful female alcohol is not a bad thing, but the abuse of alcohol is. Just because alcohol is legal does not mean it cannot cause harm and damage to your rare and precious jewel. When a person consumes alcohol in large quantities on a regular basis; that person can cause physical damage to their body. Sometime the physical damage that individual caused their body to experience will be irreversible. Listed below is some of the physical damage a person can experience from abusing alcohol.

- Brain damage
- Muscle weakness
- Anemia
- Low blood sugar
- Cirrhosis of the liver
- Pale skin
- Damage to heart muscles
- Stroke
- Low immune system
- Heart problem
- Problems with balance
- Stomach ulcers
- Blackouts
- Problem walking
- Insomnia
- Blurred vision
- Dehydration
- Kidney failure
- Coordination problems
- Fatty liver

- Tremors in hands
- Tremors in feet
- Numbness in legs
- Numbness in arms
- Tingling in arms
- Tingling in legs
- Pancreatitis
- Memory loss
- Inflammation of the stomach
- Alcohol poisoning
- Vitamin deficiencies
- Nervous System damage
- Urinary tract infection
- Destruction of brain cells
- Ulcers in the intestines
- Hyperactivity

If a person consumes alcohol in large quantities on a regular basis; that person can cause mental and emotional damage to him or herself. Listed below are some of the mental and emotion damage a person can experience from abusing alcohol.

- Increase hostility towards others
- Anxiety
- Prolong depression
- Suicidal thoughts
- Aggressive behavior towards other
- Insomnia
- Dysthymia
- Mania
- Dementia
- Panic attacks
- Schizophrenia
- Phobias

My beautiful female when a person consumes large quantities of alcohol on a regular basis that person can experience brain damage. Some of the damage that person's brain will endure because of the large quantities of alcohol is:

- Shrinkage
- Chemical alteration in the brain
- Impaired brain development (this takes place in youth)

Once a person start consuming alcohol in large quantities; on a regular basis, that person will become an Alcoholic. Now that this person is an Alcoholic there are four stages of Alcoholism he or she will go through.

First Stage of Alcoholism

In this stage the person will no longer be a social drinker. He or she will drink to escape from their problems. Basically, the person drinks to change the way he or she feels. Listed below are some of the signs of a person in the *First Stage of Alcoholism*.

- Can drink a lot of alcohol without showing signs of getting drunk
- Drinking is a way to escape problems
- Using alcohol to relax
- Consciously seeking out more alcohol in order to drink more
- Not recognizing that he or she is in the early stages of alcoholism

Second Stage of Alcoholism

In this stage the person will begin to drink earlier in the day. Now the person has to drink because he or she is dependent on it. In this stage the individual has not loss control, but he or she is in the process of losing control. Listed below are some of the signs of a person in the *Second Stage of Alcoholism*.

- Failed attempts at quitting drinking alcohol
- Sneaking drinks before he or she goes out to drink alcohol
- Denying that he or she has a drinking problem
- Blaming his or her problems on others as well as on other things
- Feeling shame from drinking
- Feeling guilt from drinking
- Frequent blackouts
- Drinking because he or she wants to alter their mood

Third Stage of Alcoholism

In this stage the person will begin to lose control over how

much alcohol he or she will consume. The individual will begin having problems with relationships with their family, friends, and co-worker. Listed below are some of the signs of a person in the *Third Stage of Alcoholism.*
- Not keeping their word or promises he or she make to people
- Aggressive behavior towards others
- Tremors
- Driving while drunk (Driving under the Influence – DUI)
- Financial problems
- Relationship problems
- Drinking alcohol first thing in the morning
- Losing control has become a normal behavior of their
- Frequent violent outburst
- No longer hang out with old friends
- Hanging out with new friends (other alcoholics)
- Making excuses for drinking in the morning
- Loss of will power
- Change in physical appearance

Fourth Stage of Alcoholism

In this stage the person will experience great loss; loss of job, loss of friends, and loss of family. Also, this individual will have to drink alcohol in order to function.

Listed below are some of the signs of a person in the *Fourth Stage of Alcoholism.*
- Extreme resentment towards others
- Extreme hostility towards others
- Shakes
- Realizing that their drinking is out of control
- Fear
- Impaired thinking
- Remorse
- Hallucination
- Feeling of pending doom
- Loss of tolerance for alcohol
- Obsessed with drinking

As you can see consuming large quantities of alcohol on a regular basis can result in you being an alcoholic. Also, it will cause damage to your rare and precious jewel. Not to mention; the psychological damage you will experience.

Plus, it can cause your kidneys, liver, and heart to not work properly. Once your kidneys, liver, and heart are unable to perform the duties they were created to do you will die.

My beautiful female there will be some people who will engage in alcohol binges. For those of you who do not know what an alcohol binge is let me explain it to you. When a person binges on alcohol he or she will consume enormous amounts of alcohol at one time. It can be done in a social gathering or by yourself.

By engaging in this behavior you will cause your rare and precious jewel to experience vitamin deficiency, dehydration, brain damage, alcohol poisoning, and death. Listed below are some of the other names used for alcohol.

- Spirits
- Booze
- Liquor
- Drank
- Moonshine
- Juice
- Brew
- Sauce
- Liquid Courage
- Cold One
- Chug
- Jack
- Poison
- Ignorant juice
- Hard stuff
- Hooch

If a person was to mix alcohol with other drugs that combination will have its own name too. Listed below are some of those combinations and their names.

- "Five Way" is Alcohol, Rohypnol, Cocaine, Heroin, and Methamphetamine

- "Fizzurp" is Champaign and Promethazine with Codeine cough syrup
- "Lochness Monster Bombs" is Jose Cuervo, Monster Energy Drink, and Promethazine with Codeine cough syrup
- "Fuzzy Sizzurp" is Peach Schnapps and Promethazine with Codeine cough syrup
- "Nati Dime" is Vodka and Dimetapp
- "Nati Dime" is Cheap Beer and Dimetapp

If you were to use any of the combination listed above you will experience side effects from the alcohol and each drug in that combination. Plus, you can die from mixing drugs with alcohol. Remember, my beautiful female; your body is a rare and precious jewel and a rare and precious jewel should be cherished and protected from harm and danger by you at all times. Consuming large quantities of alcohol on a regular basis is not an act of cherishing and protecting your rare and precious jewel.

OXYCODONE

Oxycodone is a semi-synthetic opioid analgesic narcotic. My beautiful female; the drug Oxycodone is prescribed as pain medication for sever and chronic pain. However; there are people who take this drug for recreational use. You must understand that this drug is very addictive and you should never use it to get high.

Oxycodone is a drug that mimics the same reaction in the body as Heroin. This drug causes the brain to releases high levels of the chemical *Dopamine*. Dopamine is the chemical that regulates mood, body movement, learning, and pleasure.

Some Heroin users will take Oxycodone when Heroin is not available. Since Oxycodone is time release Heroin users and other abuser of Oxycodone will crush the pill into a fine powder and snort it, they chew the pill, or they will crush the pill and dissolve it so they can bypass the time release agent in the pill.

My precious female some of the side effects a person can experience from using Oxycodone to get high are:

- Death
- Seizures
- Vomiting
- Painful breathing
- Nausea
- Headaches
- Dry mouth
- Clammy skin
- Confusion
- Fainting
- Difficulty Urinating

- Constipation
- Dizziness
- Fatigue
- Lightheadedness
- Drowsiness
- Hiccups
- Sleepiness
- Sweating
- Weakness
- Difficulty breathing
- Low blood pressure
- Impaired vision
- Anxiety
- Loss of appetite
- Tremors
- Cold skin
- Increased heart rate
- Convulsion
- Swelling of the mouth
- Heart burn
- Rashes
- Unexplained bruising
- Black stool
- Bloody stool
- Swelling of the lips
- Swelling of the tongue
- Yellowing of the skin
- Mood swings
- Tightening of the chest
- Unexplained bleeding
- Yellowing of the eyes
- Hearing loss

You should know that using Oxycodone to get high can lead to some individuals overdosing on this drug. For those of you who do not know what it mean to overdose on Oxycodone let me explain it to you. When a person overdose on Oxycodone that person has taken an amount that their heart is unable to handle. Because their heart is unable to handle the drugs he or she has taken it will stop beating. In some cases the heart explodes in the person's chest cavity. Once the heart has stopped beating or exploded in their chest cavity he or she will die.

When a person decides to stop using Oxycodone to get high that person will experience withdrawal symptoms. For those of you who do not know what withdrawal symptoms are let me explain it to you. Withdrawal symptoms are the physical and psychological changes the body will go through if an individual stops using Oxycodone (or other drugs) to get high. Listed below are some of the withdrawal symptoms that person will experience when they stop using Oxycodone.

- Depression
- Constant joint pain
- Constant muscle pain
- Diarrhea
- Vomiting
- Excessive sweating
- Excessive yawning
- Cold sweats
- Nausea
- Heart palpitation
- Coughing
- Watery eyes
- Increase heart rate
- Chills
- Craving Oxycodone

These are just a few of the withdrawal symptoms a person can experience once he or she stops using Oxycodone to get high.

My beautiful female if you are suffering from a weak kidney, liver, or heart using Oxycodone to get high can cause those organs to deteriorate even quicker. If your kidneys deteriorate it will be unable to perform the duties they were created for. If your kidneys cannot perform the duties they were created for you will die. If your liver deteriorates it will be unable to perform the duties it was created for. If your liver cannot perform the duties it was created for you will die. If your heart deteriorates it will be unable to perform the duties it was created for. If your heart cannot perform the duties it was created for you will die.

Just so you know guys who abuses Oxycodone can experience impotence, enlarge prostate, and decrease levels of testosterone.

As you can see Oxycodone can cause you physical and mental harm and in some cases death.

Listed below are some of the other names used for Oxycodone.
- Hillbilly Heroin
- OC
- Oxy
- Kickers
- Oxy 80
- Os
- Killers
- Blue
- Cotton
- Ox
- Pills
- Breeee

Remember, your body is a rare and precious jewel and a rare and precious jewel should be cherished and protected from harm and danger by you at all times. Using Oxycodone to get high is not an act of cherishing and protecting your rare and precious jewel.

MAGIC MUSHROOMS

My beautiful female you will meet people who will tell you that they use Magic Mushrooms and they are perfectly safe to use. That is not true. Let me give you some information about Magic Mushrooms. Magic Mushrooms are a psychedelic drug. The reason why they are classified as a psychedelic drug is because the Mushrooms contain *Psilocin* and *Psilocybin*. These two compounds will give you similar affects as "Tripping" on LSD.

If you were to eat any Magic Mushrooms that have become molded or the color has changed to dark brown or black you can become very ill. You will become ill because of the harmful bacteria on and in the mushrooms. If you were to eat any poisoned or molded Magic Mushrooms please seek medical attention immediately.

My beautiful female you need to realize that psychedelic drugs intensify the mental state that you were in when you took the drug. In other words if you are feeling sad, anxious, or even depressed that emotion will intensify; even if you are suppressing those emotions.

Some of the symptoms you can experience from using Magic Mushrooms to get high are:

- Stomach cramps
- Nausea
- Vomiting
- Paranoia
- Hallucinations
- Diarrhea
- Being delusional
- Loss of reality

- Audio distortion
- Visual distortion
- Recovery of suppressed memory
- Flash backs (reliving previous experiences)
- Confusion

My beautiful female another thing you will experience from using Magic Mushrooms is "Tripping". Not all "Tripping" experiences will be pleasurable. Some will be a bad "Tripping" experiences. A bad "Tripping" experience has been described as "A Living Nightmare" or "A Living Hell". The only way to get out of a bad "Tripping" experience is for the high from the Magic Mushrooms to wear off. Which mean you will have to endure the horror from your bad "Tripping" experience until your high wears off and that can be hours later. If you are wondering; is there anything you can do to speed up the bad "Tripping" experience the answer is no. There is absolutely nothing you can do to speed up the process of a bad "Tripping" experience. You will have to endure that horrific "Tripping" experience for however many hours the high last. Just so you know a tripping experience can lasted up to twelve hours.

My lovely female you will never know what "Tripping" experience you will have until you have it. You should also know that a bad "Tripping" experience can cause some people to become physically violent towards the people around them as well as themselves. In some cases people have accidentally committed suicide while "Tripping" off of Magic Mushrooms.

My beautiful female; listed below are some of the other names used for Magic Mushrooms.

- Shrooms
- Caps
- Mushrooms
- Psilocybin & Psilocyn
- Buttons
- Mushies
- Tweezes
- Liberties

- Liberty Cap
- Psilcybe Semilanceata
- Silly Putty
- God's Flesh
- Hombrecitos
- Sherms
- Simple Simon
- Capering Berries

If a person was to mix Magic Mushrooms with other drugs that combination will have its own name too. Listed below are some of those combinations and their names.

- "Flower Flipping" is Magic Mushrooms and Ecstasy
- "Hippie Flipping" is Magic Mushrooms and Ecstasy
- "Little Smoke" is Magic Mushrooms, LSD, and Marijuana
- "Sherms" is Magic Mushrooms and PCP
- "God's Flesh" is Magic Mushrooms and LSD

If you were to take any of the combinations listed above you will experience side effects from each of the drugs in that combination.

Remember, your body is a rare and precious jewel and a rare and precious jewel should be cherished and protected from harm and danger by you at all times. By using Magic Mushrooms to get high you will cause harm and damage to your rare and precious jewel.

FENTANYL

My beautiful female Fentanyl is an opioid that is used for treating Cancer and chronic pain. This pain medicine is very addictive. Fentanyl is a very potent pain medication. This drug is about 100 times more potent than Morphine, but unlike Morphine the high from Fentanyl does not last very long. Most abuser of Fentanyl will use this drug to get high because of the potency level. The abuser of Fentanyl will use this drug more often to maintain that extreme high because it does not keep you high for a long period of time. With the increase in usage it makes it easier for the abuser to become addicted to this drug. Plus, the increase in usage makes the possibility of overdosing on Fentanyl even greater.

The speed at which Fentanyl enters the bloodstream depends on if the time release agent in the pill was by passed. That is why some abusers of this narcotic would crush the pill form of Fentanyl in order to bypass the time releasing agent in the pill.

My beautiful female you can experience several different negative side effects from abusing Fentanyl to get high. Listed below are some of the negative side effects one can experience.

- Death
- Coma
- Nausea
- Vomiting
- Constipation
- Dizziness
- Drowsiness
- Headaches
- Fatigue

- Dry mouth
- Mouth sores
- Stomach pain
- Weakness
- Confusion
- Nervousness
- Hallucinations
- Diarrhea
- Anxiety
- Insomnia
- Difficulty urinating
- Itching
- Excessive sweating
- Liver damage
- Loss of appetite
- Lightheadedness
- Trouble concentrating
- Pain at injection site
- Numbness at injection site
- Irregular heart beat
- Fainting
- Seizures
- Anorexia
- Amnesia
- Hypertension
- Pale skin
- Thirst
- Rapid heart beat
- Swelling of hands
- Swelling of feet
- Addiction
- Bronchitis
- Mouth ulcers
- Indigestion
- Shortness of breath
- Weight loss

- Hypoventilation
- Flu like symptoms
- Bloating
- Feeling Full
- Heart burn
- Belching
- Difficulty breathing
- Dyspnea
- Dyspepisa

My precious female if a person was to stop abusing Fentanyl he or she will experience withdrawal symptoms. Listed below are some of the withdrawal symptoms a person can experience when he or she stop using Fentanyl to get high.

- Constipation
- Hot flashes
- Night sweats
- Loss of appetite
- Insomnia
- Anxiety
- Muscle Aches
- Joint pain
- Nausea
- Back pain
- Rapid heart beat
- Vomiting
- Chills
- Runny nose
- Eyes tearing
- Constant sneezing
- Fever
- Nervousness
- Irritability
- Weakness
- Diarrhea
- Stomach cramps
- Rapid breathing

These are just a few of the withdrawal symptoms a person can experience once he or she stops using Fentanyl to get high.

My precious female if a female was to use Fentanyl while pregnant she can cause her baby to become addicted to Fentanyl too. Once she delivers her baby he or she will go through withdrawal symptoms. Also, if she is nursing her baby while she is using Fentanyl to get high; her baby will receive Fentanyl in her breast milk. Which means her baby will be addicted to Fentanyl just like she is. If she decides to stop using Fentanyl while she is breastfeeding; her baby will go through withdrawal. This will happen because her baby is no longer receiving the very addictive drug through her breast milk.

As you can see using Fentanyl to get high while pregnant or breastfeeding your baby is a very dangerous and damaging to the baby.

Listed below are some of the other names used for Fentanyl.

- China White
- Apache
- Dance Fever
- Friends
- Great Bear
- King Ivory
- Lethal Injection
- Murder 8
- Tango & Cash
- China Girl
- Good Fellows
- Fat Albert
- China Town
- Drop Dead
- The Bomb
- Jackpot
- TNT
- Incredible Hulk

If a person was to mix Fentanyl with other drugs that combination will have its own name too. Listed below are some of

those combinations and their names.
- "Magic" is Fentanyl and Heroin
- "The Bomb" is Fentanyl and Heroin
- "Keel" is Fentanyl and Heroin
- "Poison" is Fentanyl and Heroin
- "TNT" is Fentanyl and Heroin
- "Perc-a-Pop" is flavored throat lozenges with Fentanyl on a stick
If you were to take any of the combinations listed above you will experience side effects from each of the drugs in that combination.
My beautiful female your body is a rare and precious jewel and a rare and precious jewel should be cherished and protected from harm and danger by you at all times. Using Fentanyl to get high is not an act of cherishing and protecting your rare and precious jewel

AMPHETAMINE

My beautiful female Amphetamine is a psycho-stimulant drug that triggers an increase of the chemical in the brain called *Dopamine.* Dopamine is the chemical that regulates body movement, emotions, learning, and pleasure.

This is the weakest form in the Amphetamine family. This drug mimics some of the same side effect in the body as Cocaine does. That is why people use this drug to get high. Some of the side effects a person can experience from using Amphetamines to get high are:

- Death
- Stroke
- Heart attack
- Coma
- Acne
- Jerking of the body
- Insomnia
- Fever
- Sweating
- Irritability
- Confusing
- Irregular heartbeat
- Dizziness
- Tremors
- Anxiety
- Chest pain
- Hot flashes
- Dry mouth
- Hypertension

- Nervousness
- Nausea
- Difficulty breathing
- Convulsion
- Hyperthermia
- Paranoia
- Increase blood pressure
- Increase heart rate
- Anorexia
- Dilated pupils
- Blood shot eyes
- Headaches
- Restlessness
- Itchy skin
- Blurred Vision

My beautiful female if a female uses Amphetamine to get high there is a chance that person may overdose on this drug.

When a person decides to stop using Amphetamine to get high he or she will experience withdrawal symptoms. Listed below are some of the withdrawal symptoms a person can experience.

- Fatigue
- Depression
- Mental fatigue
- Increase in appetite
- Vivid dreams
- Suicidal thoughts
- Anxiety
- Agitation
- Irritability

These are just a few of the withdrawal symptoms a person can experience once he or she stops using Amphetamine to get high. Also, the length of time that person will experience these withdrawal symptoms will vary between each individual.

My beautiful female; listed below are some of the other names used for Amphetamine.

- A

- Speed
- Whizz
- Uppers
- Christina
- French Blue
- Nugget
- Sweets
- Mollies
- Billy Whiz
- Glass
- Aimies
- Coast To Coast
- Head Drugs
- Pixies
- TR- 6's
- Pink Hearts
- Rhythm
- Snow Pallets
- Diet Pills
- Chicken Powder
- Ups
- Co-pilots
- Clear Rocks
- Black And White
- Rippers
- Bennies
- Black Beauty
- Crank
- Beans
- Benz
- Brain Tickler
- Dominoes
- Jolly Beans
- Leapers
- Football
- Hearts

- Pep Pills
- Brownies
- Oranges
- Blue Boys
- Splash
- Pink Champaign

Also, if a person was to mix Amphetamine with other drugs those combinations will have their own name too. List below are some of those combinations and their names.

- "Bombita" is Amphetamine and Heroin
- "Speedie" is Amphetamine and Ecstasy
- "Waffle Dust" is Amphetamine and Ecstasy
- "Snow Seal" is Amphetamine and Cocaine

If you were to try any of these combinations you would experience side effects from each of the drugs in that combination.

My beautiful female your body is a rare and precious jewel and a rare and precious jewel should be cherished and protected from harm and danger by you at all times. Using Amphetamine to get high will cause harm and damage to your rare and precious jewel.

SALVIA
(*Salvia Divinorum*)

My beautiful female *Salvia Divinorum* also known as *Salvia* is a psychoactive drug. This plant grows in shady and moist areas in Oaxaca Mexico, Central America, and South America. The Salvia Divinorum plant has been used by some religious groups for their religious rituals because of the hallucinogenic effect it causes them to experience.

The ingredient in Salvia that causes people to have hallucinations is *Salvinoria A*. Salvia has also been used as a home remedy to help bring relief from diarrhea, headaches, rheumatism, and anemia.

There are several ways to use this drug; you can smoke it, make a tea out of it, chew it, or eat it.

My beautiful female some people will tell you that Salvia is not dangerous, but fun because of the euphoric feeling they experienced. That is not true. There are some negative side effects you will experience from using Salvia to get high. Listed below are some of those negative side effects.

- Panic attacks
- Vivid dreams
- Anxiety
- Migraines
- Decrease in heart rate
- Increase sweating
- Increase in body temperature
- Difficulty concentrating
- Repressed memory resurfacing

- Overlapping realities
- Lack of coordination of motor skills
- Clumsiness
- Irritability
- Dizziness
- Lack of focus
- Clammy skin
- Lightheadedness
- Drowsiness
- Nausea
- Dry mouth
- Chills
- Impaired judgment
- Goosebumps
- Insomnia
- Damage to some of the receptors in the brain

My beautiful female if you use Salvia to get high you will experience what is known as the *Salvia Trip*. When experiencing the "*Salvia Trip*" you can experience six different levels which are called *S.A.L.V.I.A.*

1st Level = <u>S</u>ubtle effects

When going through the 1st level you will notice that something is different, but you cannot find the words to explain it.

2nd Level =<u>A</u>ltered

When going through the 2nd level colors will seem more vivid. Also, things will seem to be further away than what they are or closer than what they are. Your thinking will become illogical and your short term memory will become impaired.

3rd Level = <u>L</u>ight

When going through the 3rd level you will begin having light visions while your eyes are closed. You will begin seeing geometric patterns, fractal patterns, and line patterns while your eyes are closed. These images will appear two dimensional. When you open your eyes you will see some patterns, but they will vanish quickly. In this level you are not confused about reality.

4th Level = <u>V</u>ivid

When going through the 4th level your visions will become very vivid. You will experience three dimensional realistic scenes while your eyes are open. You will sometimes hear voices while experiencing these vivid visions. When you close your eyes you will fall deeper into this other reality that you see and hear. This level is unlike level three because the visions are much stronger and your eyes are open. This is the level that some of the religious groups who use Salvia for their religious rituals strive for.

5th Level = _I_mmaterial

When going through the 5th level you lose your sense of reality and you become totally involved with the visions you are having. You will also experience yourself merging with objects in your visions. When experiencing the 5th level it is impossible to function because of the severely altered state of mind you are in. This stage can be very terrifying to some people.

6th Level = _A_mnesic

When going through the 6th level your consciousness is gone. You may become immobile, you can do a lot of thrashing around, and you may display somnambulistic behavior. For those of you who do not know what Somnambulistic behavior is let me explain it to you this way. It is you being in the same state of mind as a sleep walker.

When a person reaches this level they are not consciously aware of what they are doing. Plus, the person will not feel any pain that he or she may be causing him or herself. The lack of consciousness and the inability to feel pain prevent the person from realizing that they are in the process of seriously injuring or killing him or herself and not know it. This is why the 6th level is so dangerous Also, trying to drive a vehicle at the 6th level can be very dangerous to you and the other drivers and passengers on the road. Simply because the individual is driving while interacting in that altered reality he or she is experiencing from using Salvia to get high.

Usually people can never tell you what they have experience at this level. This is a level that they did not intend to travel to. Or they simply cannot remember what took place when experiencing the 6th level because of the somnambulistic state of mind he or she was in.

As you can see using Salvia to get high is not as safe as you thought. That is why you should never use it.

Listed below are some of the other names used for Salvia.

- La Maria
- Ska Maria
- Ska Pastoria
- Hojas de Maria
- La Hembra
- Diviner's Sage
- Hierba Maria

The long term side effects of using Salvia to get high are still unknown. That mean you could be causing your rare and precious jewel damage that may be irreversible.

My beautiful female your body is a rare and precious jewel and a rare and precious jewel should be cherished and protected from harm and danger at all times by you. Using Salvia to get high can cause harm and damage to your rare and precious jewel.

PROMETHAZINE & CODEINE COUGH SYRUP

My beautiful female; there are some people who take Promethazine & Codeine Cough Syrup for recreational use (for fun). I want you to know that taking Promethazine and Codeine Cough Syrup to get high is very dangerous and it can be deadly.

For those of you who do not know much about cough syrup with Promethazine and Codeine in it let me share some information with you.

Promethazine is an Antihistamine. Promethazine is used to bring relief from:
- Itchy throat
- Water eyes
- Runny nose
- Sneezing

Listed below are some of the side effects a person can experience from taking Promethazine.
- Drowsiness
- Dry mouth
- Confusion
- Irritability
- Fatigue
- Dizziness
- Constipation
- Tightening of the chest

- Restless legs
- Pressure on the chest
- Easily agitated
- Seizures

When Promethazine is taken orally your body will absorb it in approximately 20 minutes and it can last in your body for up to six hours. In some cases it has been known to last longer than six hours.

Codeine is a narcotic that is used as pain relief. Codeine can become habit forming if you begin taking it to get high. In other words you will become addicted to Codeine.

Listed below are some of the side effects a person can experience from using Codeine to get high.

- Seizures
- Kidney damage
- Liver damage
- Difficulty breathing
- Swelling of the tongue
- Dizziness
- Constipation
- Sweating
- A rash
- Itching
- Vomiting
- Stomach pain
- Nausea
- Drowsiness
- Difficulty urination
- Mood swings
- Confusion
- Agitation
- Hallucinations
- Irrational thoughts
- Erratic behavior
- Lightheadedness
- Slow heart rate

- Swollen lips
- Swelling of the face
- Fainting
- Shallow breathing
- Swelling of the throat
- Loss of coordination
- Blurred vision
- Stomach bleeding
- Tremors
- Becoming disoriented
- Headaches
- Insomnia
- Restlessness
- Stiffness
- Chest pain
- Unusual bruising
- Chills

When a person takes cough syrup with Promethazine and Codeine to get high that person can experience side effects from both of the drugs in the cough syrup.

If the person began having complication from abusing this cough syrup and he or she does not seek medical treatment there is a chance that person may die.

My beautiful female when a person decides to stop using Promethazine and Codeine Cough Syrup to get high that individual will experience withdrawal symptoms. For those of you who do not know what withdrawal symptoms are let me explain it to you. Withdrawal symptoms are the different physical and psychological changes the body will go through when a person stops using Promethazine and Codeine Cough Syrup (or other drugs) to get high.

Listed below are some of the withdrawal symptoms you can experience from using Promethazine and Codeine Cough Syrup to get high.

- Anxiety
- Fever

- Diarrhea
- Nausea
- Restless legs
- Vomiting
- Insomnia
- Pain
- Achy muscles

These are just a few of the withdrawal symptoms a person can experience once he or she stops using Promethazine and Codeine Cough Syrup to get high.

Listed below are some of the other names used for Promethazine and Codeine Cough Syrup when it is mixed with sprite, kool aide, or any other liquid that a person choose to mix with the cough syrup. As well as some of the names that is used when Jolly Ranchers are added to the mixtures.

- Sizzurp
- Syrup
- Screw Juice
- Drank
- Purple Drank
- Fizzy Sizzurp
- Promo
- Nemo
- Purple Stuff
- Fizzurp
- Sizzy
- SPM
- Lean
- Purple Magic
- Skeet Chase
- Oil
- Barre
- Purp
- Texas Tea
- Pink Sprite
- Purple Sprite

- Purple

My beautiful female using cough syrup with Promethazine and Codeine in it to get high is not a very smart or safe thing to do. You can cause your body a lot of damage and harm from using Promethazine and Codeine Cough Syrup to get high. You should also know that there is a chance that you may die from using this cough syrup to get high.

Remember, your body is a rare and precious jewel and a rare and precious jewel should be cherished and protected from harm and danger by you at all times. Using cough syrup with Promethazine and Codeine in it to get high is not an act of cherishing and protecting your rare and precious jewel.

INHALANTS

My precious female; there are some people who use inhalants to get high. These individuals choose inhalants because they are easily available and very cheap. For those of you who do not know what products are considered inhalants; let me tell you what some of them are:

- Household cleaning products
- Cans of spray paint
- Hair spray
- Gasoline
- Furniture polish
- Paint thinner
- Inhalers
- Markers
- Paint remover
- Breath spray
- Nail polish remover
- Glue
- Felt Pens
- Felt tip markers
- Varnish
- High lighters
- Vegetable spray
- Nail polish

These are just a few of the many items that are used as inhalants. My beautiful female inhalants can be used several different ways to get high. Listed below are the different ways people use inhalants to get high.

1st way - Bagging

Bagging is when an individual spray the inhalant in a plastic bag and place the plastic bag over their head. Then the individual will hold the bottom of the plastic bag closed around their neck and inhale the toxic fumes.

2nd way - Sniffing

Sniffing is when a person would sniff things like glue, felt pens, felt markers, highlighters, finger nail polish, finger nail polish remover, and gasoline to get high. Just so you know there are many more items used for sniffing.

3rd way - Huffing

Huffing is when an individual soak a rag with chemicals and hold it up to their nose and inhale the fumes. Sometimes the chemical soaked rag is placed in the person mouth and the individual will inhale the fumes that way.

My beautiful female by engaging in any of the three ways listed above to get high you can cause damage to your rare and precious jewel. Listed below are some of the short term side effects a person can experience from using inhalants to get high.

- Hallucinations
- Paranoia
- Seizures
- Loss of consciousness
- Nausea
- Vomiting
- Becoming delusional
- Headaches
- Nose bleeds
- Bad breath
- Mood swings
- Muscle weakness
- Chemical burns on the lips
- Glossy eyes
- Sweating
- Memory loss
- Coughing
- Abdominal pain

- Numbness
- Tingling in the hands
- Tingling in the feet
- Loss of appetite
- Chemical burns on the face
- Loss of coordination
- Impaired thinking
- Red eyes
- Fatigue
- Dizziness
- Limb spasm
- Slurred speech
- Irritability
- Dilated pupils
- Sores on and around the mouth
- Sores on and around the nose
- Irregular heart beat
Some of the long term side effects a person can experience from using inhalants to get high are listed below.
- Death
- Brain damage
- Heart attack
- Depression
- Paranoia
- Kidney damage
- Liver damage
- Lung damage
- Heart damage
- Muscle damage
- Nerve damage
- Loss of vision
- Loss of hearing
- Anxiety
- Bone marrow diseases
- Limb spasm
My beautiful female; once you damage your lungs from using

inhalants it is not reversible. If your lungs are not able to perform the duties they were created to do you can and will die. This is why you should never use inhalants to get high.

When a person decides to stop using inhalants to get high he or she will experience withdrawal symptoms. For those of you who do not know what withdrawal symptoms are let me explain it to you. Withdrawal symptoms are the different physical and psychological changes the body will go through if an individual stops using Inhalants to get high. Listed below are some of the withdrawal symptoms he or she will experience.

- Paranoia
- Suicidal thoughts
- Depression
- Headaches
- Chills
- Sweating
- Loss of appetite
- Mood swings
- Craving the inhalants

My beautiful female; there are four different types of inhalants that pre-teens, teenagers, young adults, and even older adults use to get high.

The First Type Of Inhalant Is Solvents

For those of you who do not know what a solvent is let me explain it to you. A Solvent is a substance that is capable of dissolving another substance. The products that will fall under Solvents are:

- Lighter fluid
- Kerosene
- Toxic Markers
- Gasoline
- Correction fluid
- Paint
- Paint thinner
- Pure toluene

The Second Type Of Inhalant Is Gases

For those of you who do not know what gas is let me explain it to you. Gas is the fluid form of a substance in which it can expand indefinitely and completely fill its container. This substance is neither liquid nor solid; it is a vapor.

The products that will fall under Gas are:

- Butane
- Nitrous Oxide
- Propane
- Helium

The Third Type Of Inhalant Is Aerosol

For those of you who do not know what Aerosol is let me explain it to you. Aerosol is a substance enclosed under pressure and able to be released as a fine spray by means of a propellant gas. The products that will fall under Aerosols are:

- Spray paint
- Deodorant
- Room spray
- Hair spray
- Fabric protector
- Vegetable cooking spray

The Fourth Type Of Inhalant Is Nitrate

For those of you who do not know what Nitrate is let me explain it to you. Nitrate is the univalent radical No3 or a compound containing it as a salt or ester of Nitric acid. The products that will fall under Nitrate are:

- Amyl
- Butyl

My beautiful female I want you to know that there are four ways you can die from using inhalants to get high.

1st Way - Sudden Sniffing Death

When this happen the individual's heart rate will increase at an alarming rate and then their heart will suddenly stop beating. This is known as Cardiac Arrest or simply that person had a heart attack.

2nd Way - Asphyxia

When this happen the oxygen in the individual's lungs is replaced with the toxic fumes he or she has been inhaling. Once the oxygen is replaced with the toxic fumes the individual will stop breathing. When the individual stop breathing he or she will die.

3rd Way - Suffocation

This will take place when the individual spray inhalants in a plastic bag and place the plastic bag over their head. By doing this the individual will cut off the oxygen that their brain needs in order to function properly. If the individual's brain is not able to get oxygenized blood that person will suffocate. Plus, the toxic fumes he or she is breathing will cause the oxygen to leave even quicker.

4th Way - Suicide

When an individual uses inhalant to get high that person can become psychologically dependent on them. When that person is unable to use inhalants to get high it can lead to depression. Because of the depression that individual will kill himself or herself because he or she is unable to handle the depress feelings that he or she is having.

As you can see using inhalants to get high is just as dangerous as using any other drug. That is why you should never use inhalants to get high.

My beautiful female, listed below are some of the other names used for inhalants.

- Climax
- Bullet Bolt
- Medusa
- Moon Gas
- Oz
- Pearl
- Toilet Water
- Whippets
- Satan's Secret
- Snappers
- Rush
- Honey Oil

- Thrust
- Shoot The Breeze
- Hardware
- Aroma Of Men
- Boppers
- Bang
- Whiteout
- Poor Man's Pot
- Spray Snot Ball
- Bolt
- Texas Shoe Shine
- Hippie Crack
- Heart On
- Buzz Bomb
- Chroming
- Quick Silver
- Air Blast
- Ames
- Discorama
- Aimies
- Highball
- Amys

My precious one your body is a rare and precious jewel and a rare and precious jewel should be cherished and protected from harm and danger at all time by you. Using inhalants to get high will cause your rare and precious jewel harm and damage.

BATH SALT

My beautiful female you probably heard people talking about using "Bath Salt" to get high. For those of you who do not know what "Bath Salt" is let me explain it to you. First of all; the drug "Bath Salt" is not the same bath salt that you put in your bath water. This "Bath Salt" is a drug that you snort, smoke, swallow, or inject into your veins to get high.

This drug contains *Mephedrone* and *Methylenedioxypyrovalerone* (MDPV) along with other chemicals. "Bath Salt" has been reported as having some of the same negative effects on the body as Methamphetamine, LSD, and PCP.

If an individual was to use "Bath Salt" to get high these are some of the negative side effects that person can experience.
- Death
- Extreme paranoia
- Hallucinations
- Seizures
- Impaired short term memory
- Rapid heartbeat
- Anxiety
- Panic attacks
- Depression
- Chest pain
- Hypertension
- Craving more "Bath Salt"
- High blood pressure
- Suicidal thoughts
- Irritability
- Dizziness

- Teeth grinding
- Headaches
- Erratic behavior
- Hyperthermia
- Renal failure
- Nose bleeds (if snorted)
- Pain in nasal cavity (if snorted)
- Circulatory problems
- Mood swings
- Violent behavior
- Having psychotic episodes
- Easily agitated
- Feeling invincible (delusional)
- Feeling like you have super human strength (delusional)
- Feeling like you can fly (delusional)

This drug causes some people to become delusional and believe they can do things like flying, being invincible, or acquiring super human strength. Because these individuals are delusional they will do things that will cause them to accidentally kill themselves.

My beautiful female you need to know that this drug is very addictive. There have been cases where individuals will crave the drug while in the emergency room. Sometime the patient would have to be sedated because of the psychotic behavior they are displaying.

As of now the doctors and scientist do not know the long term damage "Bath Salt" will cause the body. Which means the people who are using "Bath Salt" to get high could be causing irreversible damage to their rare and precious jewel.

Listed below are some of the other names used for "Bath Salt".

- MCAT
- Drone
- Meow
- Bubbles
- Ivory Wave
- Purple Wave

- Vanilla Sky
- IW
- Ivory Coast
- Blizzard
- Blue Silk
- Charge+
- Stardust
- White Dove
- White Knight
- White Lightening
- Bliss
- Hurricane Charlie
- Red Dove

As you can see using "Bath Salt" to get high is very dangerous and harmful to the body. Plus, the long term side effects this drug will have on the body and mind is not know as of yet which makes Bath salt even more dangerous.

My beautiful female your body is a rare and precious jewel and a rare and precious jewel should be cherished and protected from harm and danger by you at all times. Using "Bath Salt" to get high is not how you cherish and protect your rare and precious jewel from harm and danger.

K2

(Synthetic Cannabis)

K2 is an herb and chemical mixture that is sold as Herbal Incense, but it is not being used as incense. This drug is being used as a substitution for Marijuana. Listed below are some of the reasons why K2 is being substituted for Marijuana.

- The chemicals in K2 mimic the same side effects as THC in Marijuana.
- K2 is legal to purchase.
- K2 is easily accessible.
- K2 is more potent than Marijuana.

K2 or "Fake Weed" as some people call it; is not a safe product for people to smoke. Some people may think it is safe to smoke because it is legal, but that is not true. The reason why K2 is legal is because the chemicals that are used to make K2 are not banned in the United States per the FDA (Food and Drug Administration).

Some of those chemicals and synthetic Cannabinoids that are used in making K2 are: Cannabicyclohexanol, JWH-073, JWH-018, and HU210. Just so you know some states have made these Cannabinoids illegal: JWH-20, JWH-073, CP-47, and Cannabicyclohexanol.

This action was taken to ban the sale of "Herbal Incense" in their state. Those Cannabinoids have the potential to be extremely harmful to people who use them to get high. Also, it can cause the individual who had taken them to become a danger to society.

Because some states have made those four chemicals illegal

manufacturers of K2 would change the chemicals they use to manufacture K2. Once the chemicals were changed it allow K2 to be sold in those states legally even though it is a dangerous drug. Because of the constant changes in the chemicals several states have found it difficult to classify K2 as an illegal drug.

My beautiful young female some of the side effects a person can experience from using K2 to get high are:

- Extreme Paranoid
- Horrific hallucinations
- Strong desire to kill others
- Strong desire to kill oneself
- Mental disturbances
- Extreme feelings of pending doom
- Dizziness
- Confusion
- Illogical thinking
- Seizures
- Convulsion
- Audible Hallucination
- Fear
- Difficulty breathing
- Sweating
- No concept of time
- No concept or reality
- Unconsciousness
- Experiencing side effect after discontinued use of K2

You must understand that the long term side effects of K2 are unknown. Which means you may be causing harm and damage to your body that may be irreversible.

Listed below are other names and brand names used for "fake Weed".

- K2
- K3
- K4
- Spice
- K Royal

- Spike 99 Ultra
- 2010
- Smoke
- Genie
- Ocean Blue
- Hush
- Mystery
- Buzz
- Pulse
- Pot-pourri
- Earthquake
- Serenity
- Stinger
- Oyster
- Dragon Spice
- Zombie World
- G Four
- Shanti Spice
- Chronic Spice
- XTREME Spice
- Samurai Spice
- Midnight Chill
- Spicylicious
- Woodstock
- Who Dat
- Scooby Snacks
- Purple Haze
- Kush

My lovely female your body is a rare and precious jewel and a rare and precious jewel is meant to be cherished and protected from harm and danger by you at all times. Using K2 to get high will cause harm and damage to your rare and precious jewel. Plus, it may cause harm and damage to your body that may be irreversible. Using drugs that can cause irreversible damage to your rare and precious jewel is not an act of cherishing and protecting your rare and precious jewel.

MESCALINE

My beautiful female Mescaline is a psychedelic alkaloid drug. This drug is brown in color and it comes from the crown of the Mexican Cactus Peyote Plant. Some religious groups would use Mescaline as a part of their religious rituals because of the hallucinogenic effects of the drugs. Mescaline is not as safe as people will have you to believe. That is why you should not use it to get high. Listed below are some of the short term side effects a person can experience from using Mescaline to get high.

- Increase heart rate
- Nausea
- Convulsion
- Unconsciousness
- Headaches
- Dizziness
- Vomiting
- Irrational though processing
- Fear of pending doom
- Distorted vision
- Distorted audio
- Pupil dilation
- Excessive sweating
- Paranoia
- Muscle weakness
- Clumsiness
- Lack of balance
- Fatigue
- Queasiness
- Difficulty breathing

- Tightening of muscles in the neck
- Tightening of muscles in the face
- Irrational thinking

Not only will that person experience short term side effects he or she will experience long term side effects too. List below are some of the long term side effects a person can experience from using Mescaline to get high.

- Heart failure
- Death
- Respiratory failure
- Systolic blood pressure
- Depression
- Anxiety
- Fear of pending doom
- Paranoia
- Difficulty breathing

As you can see using Mescaline to get high can be very damaging to you physically and mentally. Plus, it can kill you.

Another thing a person may experience from using Mescaline to get high is overdosing on it. For those of you who do not know what it means to overdose on Mescaline (or other drugs) let me explain it to you. When an individual overdose on drugs he or she has taken an amount that their heart is unable to handle. Because their heart is unable to handle the drugs he or she has taken it will stop beating. In some cases the heart explodes in the person's chest cavity. Once that person's heart stops beating or exploded in their chest cavity he or she will die.

My beautiful female; listed below are some of the other names used for Mescaline.

- Buttons
- Moon
- Cactus
- Beans
- Cactus Buttons
- Cactus Head
- Chief

- Mesc
- Mescal
- Topi
- Peyote Button
- San Pedro
- Mescap
- Mese
- Mezc

If a person was to combine Mescaline with other drugs those combinations will have their own name as well. List below are some of those combinations and their names.

- "Love Tripping" is Mescaline and Ecstasy
- "Love Flipping" is Mescaline and Ecstasy
- "Snackies" is Mescaline and pure Ecstasy

If you were to take any of the combinations listed above you will experience side effects from each of the drugs in that combination.

My beautiful female your body is a rare and precious jewel and a rare and precious jewel should be cherished and protected from harm and danger by you at all times. By using Mescaline to get high you will cause harm and damage to your rare and precious jewel.

XANAX

My beautiful female Xanax is a drug that is used for treating someone who suffers from panic disorders or anxiety. Xanax is a *Benzodiazepines* drug. This drug affects the neurotransmitter in the Central Nervous System (CNS) called *Gamma Amino-Butyric Acid (GABA)*. In other words Xanax acts as a sedative for the Central Nervous System. Some people like to use Xanax to get high because they like the relaxed feeling that the drug causes them to experience.

Using Xanax to get high can lead to you experiencing negative side effects. Listed below are some of the negative side effects a person may experience from using Xanax to get high.

- Suicidal thoughts
- Depression
- Hallucinations
- Rage
- Confusion
- Lightheadedness
- Fatigue
- Dry mouth
- Seizures
- Headache
- Change in sex drive
- Fever
- Anterograde amnesia
- Difficulty breathing
- Swelling of the tongue
- Swelling of the face
- Swelling of the lips

- Change in sex drive
- Increase in saliva
- Slurred speech
- Skin rashes
- Constipation
- Drowsiness
- Dizziness
- Lack of coordination
- Aggression
- Mania
- Respiratory problems
- Jaundice
- Hyperactivity
- Cold and clammy hands
- Lack of focus
- Restlessness
- Tremors
- Twitching
- Hostility
- Hives
- Tightening to the chest
- Mood swings
- Blurred vision
- Burning in the chest
- Numbness
- Fainting
- Irregular heart beat
- Loss of muscle control
- Irregular menstrual cycle
- Decrease in urination
- Itching
- Blistering skin
- Dark color urine

My beautiful female if you start taking Xanax to get high your body will become dependent on it. In other words your body will need to have Xanax in order for you to be able to function.

If an individual decides to stop using Xanax to get high he or she will have to be weaned off this drug. If he or she decides to abruptly stop using Xanax that person will experience psychological changes. Those psychological changes will cause his or her behavior to become so erratic and out of control that he or she may cause harm to him or herself or the people around them. In some case that erratic behavior has led to accidental deaths.

When a person stops using Xanax to get high that person will experience withdrawal symptoms. Listed below are some of the withdrawal symptoms a person can experience when he or she stop using Xanax to get high.

- Paranoia
- Seizures
- Panic attacks
- Anxiety
- Confusion
- Depression
- Vomiting
- Nausea
- Diarrhea
- Dizziness
- Fear
- Fever
- Hallucinations
- Heart palpitation
- Muscle spasm
- Headaches
- Mood swings
- Sensitivity to light
- Sensitivity to sounds
- Abdominal cramps
- Blurred vision
- Insomnia
- Memory loss
- Rapid heartbeat

- Sweating
- Restlessness
- Agitation
- Convulsions
- Tremors

These are just a few of the withdrawal symptoms an individual can experience once he or she stops using Xanax to get high.

My beautiful female if you use Xanax while you are pregnant you will cause your baby to be addicted to Xanax too. Once your baby is born he or she will go through withdrawal symptoms because he or she is no longer receiving the drug Xanax.

Listed below are some of the different brand names used for Xanax in the United States.

- Danox
- Krama
- Zolam
- Alzam
- Neupax
- Grifoalpram
- Prenadona
- Tranax
- Stresnil
- Docalprazo
- Tensium Gastric
- Zotran
- Alprazomed
- Saturnil
- Xanax XR
- Alprocontin
- Topazolam
- Xanacine
- Tafil
- Pazolam
- Restyl Plus
- Amziax
- PTA

- Anzilum
- Renax
- Marzolam
- Fludep Plus
- Anax
- Helex
- Euciton Stress
- Adax
- Psicosedol
- Frontin
- Tranquinal Soma
- Alcelam
- Xanor
- Zopax
- Becede
- Calmax
- Prazam
- Xycalm
- Alnax
- Siampraxol
- Sidoma
- Trankimazin
- Xiemed
- Alprax
- Tricalma
-Restyl Forte
- Pacyl
- Bestrol
- Ansielix
- Farmapram
- Niravam
- Zacetin
- Xanagir
- Alpravecs
- Neurol
- Prinox

- Mialin
- Emeral
- Alplax
- Gerax
- Alprax
- Frontal
- Kalma
- Sanerva
- Unilan
- Valeans
- Tensium
- Retan
- Nalion
- Cassadan
- Alpralid
- Apo-Alprax
- Calmo
- Farmapram
- Azor
- Thiprazolan
- Medronal
- Dizolam

My beautiful female some of the street names used for Xanax is:
- Sticks
- Handlebars
- Bars
- Stikalix
- Z-Bars
- Yellow Boys
- Bicycle Parts
- White Boys
- White Girls
- Footballs
- School Bus

As you can see using Xanax to get high is very dangerous to you physically and mentally.

Lora McDuffie

My beautiful female you must realize that your body is a rare and precious jewel and a rare and precious jewel is meant to be cherished and protected from harm and danger by you at all times. Using Xanax to get high is not an act of cherishing and protecting your rare and precious jewel.

DATING

My beautiful female going out on dates can be a very exciting and wonderful experience. It can also be a very dangerous experience. That is why it is very important that you know how to stay safe while dating. By knowing how to stay safety while dating you can keep the dating experience as exciting and wonderful as it can be as well as safe. Listed below are several things you should do in order to stay safe while dating.

Safety Tips

1st Safety Tip – Always keep some money with you when you go on your date.
If the guy tries to equate that you have to have sex with him because he is spending his money on you; you are able to pay for your own purchase. Just so you know you are not obligated to have sex with a guy just because he buys you something; no matter if it was something expensive or inexpensive.
Also, if the guy you are on a date with becomes irate, disrespectful, drunk, high, or unsafe to be with you are able to take a taxi or public transportation to get back home.

2nd Safety Tip – Always keep a charged cell phone with you on your date.
By having a charged cell phone you are able to contact the police or Emergency Medical Services (EMS) if needed. Plus, you may need to call someone to come and pick you up because your date has become intoxicated, high on drug, irate, disrespectful, or just unsafe to be with.

3rd Safety Tip – Do not go to the guy's house for your date.
My beautiful female it is much easier for the guy to convince you to do something you do not want to do if you are at his house. Being at the guy's house can remove the comfort and safety you would have felt if you would have been in a public place, at home, or at a relative's house. Plus, there is a chance that his parents may not be home and he forces you to have sex with him. Just so you know if the guy you are on a date with forces you to have sex with him that is called *Date Rape*. If this was to ever happen to you please tell your parents and file a police report against your attacker.

4th Safety Tip – Do not drink alcohol while on your date.
If you were to drink any alcohol even a little alcohol it can impair your judgment. Alcohol will cause you to involuntarily lower your guard and do things you normally would not do. One thing you should know is that females have a lower level of tolerance for alcohol than males. In other words it takes less alcohol to get a female drunk and intoxicated than it does a male.
5th Safety Tip – If you are drinking a drink (any beverage) and you leave your drink do not go back and drink that drink.
If your drink was left unattended there could be a chance that someone put a Date Rape Drug, a tranquilizer, a sedative, Ketamine, or any other debilitating drug in your drink. These drugs are used to make you incoherent and nonresponsive to what is going on around you or to you. When a Date Rape Drug, a tranquilizer, a sedative, Ketamine, or any other debilitating drug is used on you there is nothing good that can come out of that situation.
The guys who spike females drinks usually plans on raping, robbing, abducting, or murdering the female whose drink he has spiked. Sometime the guy may do all four things to his victim.
When you drink a spike drink you will remember what happen hours before you had taken the drug and after the drug has worn off. In some cases you may be aware of what is going on, but you are unable to resist or fight back because of the drug or the

amount that was used on you.

My beautiful female you need to understand that even though you may not remember what had taken place or you were unable to resist or fight back this is still considered as rape. The fact that this guy drugged you in order for you to have sex with him without your permission makes it rape. That is why if you did not see the person make your drink or you left your drink unattended you should not drink that drink. Better safe than sorry.

6th Safety Tip – Make sure your parents know the full name (not just his nick name) and the phone number of the guy you are going out on a date with.

By providing this information to your parents or someone else if anything was to happen to you they will have some information to give to the police.

7th Safety Tip – Always have several conversations with the guy via cell phone before going out on a date with him.

By talking to the guy on the phone you will get a chance to witness the guy's character. For instance; is he a guy who is obsessed with having sex, is he a guy who is possessive, or is he a guy who has a bad temper?

If the guy you are talking to on the phone possesses some of the characteristics you find undesirable you know not to go out on a date with him. Or you may find out that the guy is really cool and you both like doing some of the same things. If this is the case by all means go out and enjoy your date.

My beautiful female I want you to understand that it is very easy to hide who you are when you are chatting with someone via Facebook or any other social media outlet. That is why it is very important to spend some time talking to them on the phone before agreeing to go out on a date with them. By talking to the guy on the phone you will be able to pick up on agitation and rage through the tone of their voice.

8th Safety Tip – Always introduce the guy to your
family before going out on a date with him.
The adults in your family will be able to tell if he is a good guy,
if he is trouble and you should leave him alone, or if he is only
dating you because he wants to have sex with you. Plus, your
family will know what the guy looks like in case something was
to happen to you.

9th Safety Tip – Do not wear very revealing
and sexy clothes on your date.
Wearing very revealing and sexy clothes can give the guy you
are on your date with the wrong impression about you. Some
guys will assume that the very revealing and sexy clothes you
are wearing is an invitation to have sex. Sometimes a guy may
pursue you very aggressively to have sex with him because of
the very revealing and sexy clothes you are wearing. In some
cases the guy you are on a date with may force you to have sex
with him because he refuses to accept you saying No to sex because of the very revealing and sexy clothes you are wearing.
My beautiful female; just so you know if the guy you are on a
date with forces you to have sex with him that is called *Date
Rape.* If this was to ever happen to you please tell your parents
and file a police report against your attacker. I want you to
understand that just because you have on sexy and revealing
clothes does not give a guy the right to rape you. One way to
avoid having this happen to you is to not wear very revealing
and sexy clothes on your date; wear really cute clothes that
compliment your figure.

10th Safety Tip – Do not get high on your date.
Getting high will impair your judgment and it will cause you to
do thing that you will normally not do. You need to understand
that your first time doing drugs may be your last time doing
drugs because you have over dosed on the drugs you were taking. Plus, you may go into cardiac arrest from the drug you had
taken. You may even develop brain damage from the drugs you

have taken.

11th Safety Tip – Do not talk about sex on your date.
Some guys consider sexual conversation as an invitation for sex. In some cases the guy you are out on your date with may try to force you to have sex with him because of the sexual conversation you both were having. Some of the guys may rape you because they refuse to accept you saying No to sex because of the sexual conversation you both were having. My beautiful female if this was to happen to you please tell your parents and file a police report against your attacker. What he did to you was wrong and you did not deserve to be rape because of the sexual conversation you both were having. By the way this is known as *Date Rape* and date rape is against the law.

12th Safety Tip – When you live on your own and you are going out on a date always make sure you let someone know when, where, and who you are going out on a date with.
By doing this it will always keep someone familiar with what you are doing. Plus, if anything was to happen to you there will be someone to assist the police.

13th Safety Tip – Do not do anything that makes you uncomfortable.
By not doing things that makes you uncomfortable you will be able to avoid doing thing you really do not want to do. Plus, it will keep you from being in undesirable situations.

ABUSE

Anything that is harmful, injurious, or offensive. Abuse also includes excessive and wrongful misuse of anything. There are several major types of abuse: physical, sexual, emotional, and substance abuse.

PHYSICAL ABUSE

My beautiful female you are a wonderful gift to the world and any guy you date should feel honored that you have agreed to go out on a date with him. Dating someone who does not see your true value can lead to you facing many undesirable situations. One undesirable situation you should know about is physical abuse.

My beautiful female; you should know that physical abuse can be done many different ways. Physical abuse is punching someone to control them. Physical abuse is pushing and shoving someone to control them. Physical abuse is slapping someone to control them. Physical abuse is slamming someone into walls to control them. Physical abuse is pulling someone around by their hair to control them. Physical abuse is throwing things at someone to control them. Physical abuse is grabbing someone by their neck to control them. Physical abuse is pushing someone down the stairs to control them. Physical abuse is kicking someone to control them. Physical abuse is throwing someone into and over furniture to control them. Physical abuse is dragging someone around by their legs and arms to control them. Physical abuse is slamming someone on to the floor to control them. Physical abuse is slamming someone into to lockers to control them. Physical abuse is shaking someone franticly to control them. Physical abuse is bending someone's fingers back to control them. As you can see physical abuse can be done many different ways.

My precious female there is never a good reason for the guy you are dating to be physically abusive towards you.

Physical abuse should never be an acceptable behavior from a guy you are dating, or in a relationship with, or even married to; no one has the right to be physically abusive towards you.

My Lovely female you should never make excuses for why a guy is physically abusive towards you. There is never a good reason for the guy you are dating or married to; to physically abuse to you. Your body is a rare and precious jewel and a rare and precious jewel should be cherished and protected; not physically abused.

If the guy you are dating is beating on you he does not value you and he does not see how special you are. Staying in a relationship or dating someone that is physically abusive can lead to you having physical injuries and even internal injuries. Sometimes those injuries can lead to your death. Or he can just beat you to death.

What you need to understand my beautiful female is that dating should be a wonderful and exciting experience not a horrible, terrifying, and abusive experience.

When you date a guy who is physically abusive the abuse usually continues and gets worse.

I want you to know that not all acts of physical abuse leaves scars on your body. Just because some of the things that are done to you do not leave a scar on your body does not mean it is not physical abuse. If your abuser held a pillow over your face to control you; that would not leave a scar on you, but that is still physical abuse. If your abuser drugged you around by your legs and arms to control you; that would not leave a scar on you, but that is still physical abuse. If your abuser pulled your hair to control you; that would not leave a scar on you, but that is still physical abuse. If your abuser threw water in your face to control you, that would not leave a scar on you, but that is still physical abuse. If your abuser punched you in the stomach to control you; that would not leave a scar on you, but that is still physical abuse. If your abuser kicked you in the stomach to control you; that would not leave a scar on you, but that is still physical abuse. If your abuser punched you in your breast to control you; that would not leave a scar on you, but that is still physical abuse. If your abuser kicked you in your derriere to control you; that would not leave a scar on you, but that is still physical abuse. If your abuser punched you in your side to control you; that would not leave a scar on you, but that is still physical abuse. If your abuser bent your arm behind your back to control you; that would not leave a scar on you, but that is still physical abuse. If your abuser bent your fingers back to control you; that would not leave a scar on you, but that is still physical abuse. If your abuser hit you in your head to control you; that would not leave a scar on you, but that is still physical abuse. If your abuser spit saliva in your face to control you; that would not leave a scar on you, but that is still physical abuse. As you can see an abuser can physically abuse you and not leave scars on your body.

I want you to know my beautiful female that physical abuse is physical abuse whether it leaves a scar on your body or not.

If you are being physically abused by a guy you are dating that is his way of controlling you. He is controlling you through fear and violence.

My beautiful female you are a very courageous person and if someone is physically abusive towards you I want you to tell someone and get out of that relationship or stop dating that guy. I want you to get out of that situation before your abuser seriously injures you or possibly beat you to death. If your abuser has threatened you; you should take his threats seriously and file a Personal Protection Order (PPO) against your attacker. That way he will not be allowed to come near you and if he does he can be arrested and taken to jail.

My beautiful female you should know that an abuser will come up with many excuses as to why he is physically abusive towards you. Listed below are some of the excuses your abuser will use.

1st Excuse – You see what you made me do to you?

2nd Excuse – If you would just do what I ask I won't have to do this.

3rd Excuse – If you would just shut up none of this would have ever happened.

4th Excuse – I do not know what came over me.

5th Excuse – You know when I see you talking to other guys it make me crazy.

6th Excuse – You know I do not like it when you do not answer my calls.

7th Excuse – Where were you? You know how I get when I cannot find you.

8th Excuse – I'm sorry. I will never hit you again.

9th Excuse – I did not want to hit you, but you made me do it.

10th Excuse – I really do not want to do this, but you just will not do right.

11th Excuse – You never learn

12th Excuse – Look what you made me do to you

13th Excuse – If you would quit talking back I would not have to hit you.

14th Excuse – I'm sorry. I'm just so stressed.

15th Excuse – I see I'm going to have to teach you a lesson about disrespecting me.

16th Excuse – You think I'm playing with you? Let me show you how serious I am.

17th Excuse – You're going to ignore me?

18th Excuse – are you cheating on me?

19th Excuse – If you would quit lying I would not have to do this.

20th Excuse – I don't want to do this, but it's for your own good.

21st Excuse – I do not like having to do this, but this is the only way you gone learn.

Guys who are physically abusive will say it is your fault why they would abuse you. They rarely see that they abuse you because they choose to. You need to realize that no matter what you do, what you say, or even who you talk to does not give anyone the right to physically abuse you. You are a precious gift and you are meant to be loved and cherished not beaten. Any guy that beats on you does not deserve someone as special as you.

If you have to file a Personal Protection Order (PPO) against your abuser do not feel bad about it. PPO's were created to protect people from individuals who will harm them and your abuser is harming you.

When you file your PPO against your abuser be sure to let the officer know that you do not feel safe and you know your abuser will harm you. You must make it clear to the officer that you are fearful of this person. Whatever you do; do not down play the harm your abuser have caused you in the past and will cause you in the future.

My beautiful female you probably are feeling embarrassed and ashamed about being abused by the guy you are dating. You should not feel that way. Being physically abused is nothing you should be embarrassed and ashamed of. The person who is abusing you should feel embarrassed and ashamed because he is beating on you to control you.

You on the other hand need to understand that it is ok to leave your abusive boyfriend. You do not have to continue dating someone who is physically abusive towards you. When the guy you are dating is physically abusive towards you; you should stop dating that guy. The person you date should uplift and encourage you not beat on you.

My precious female I want you to know that it is ok to have love in your heart for someone and not be around that person. Your heart is going to feel what it feels, but it is not ok for the person you love to physically abuse you. I want you to know that it is ok to stop dealing with someone you love because he is causing you harm and pain. You have to love yourself just as much as you love the person abusing you. When you love yourself you would do any and everything to protect yourself from harm and danger. If the guy you are dating is causing you harm and danger that mean you have to protect yourself from him. If leaving him is the only way you can protect yourself from him that is what you have to do.

My beautiful female I want you to remember that you are a precious gift and a precious gift is meant to be loved and cherished and not beaten.

If you are dating a guy who is physically abusive and you do not want to give up on what you have because things use to be so good in the beginning; you are deceiving yourself. What you need to understand is that in the beginning when you were dating he had to be a very sweet guy to convince you that he was a good guy and not a monster. By him being really sweet to you in the beginning it allowed you to see what he is capable of as well as distort who he really is. Even though this guy may have been very sweet to you in the past you need to still pay attention to his behavior and actions towards you now. Do not let the kindness that your abusive boyfriend showed you in the beginning blind you into staying in an abusive relationship. Do not allow the kindness that a guy showed you in the past influence you to stay in an abusive relationship. Staying in a physically abusive relationship; because the guy use to be nice and sweet can lead to you being seriously injured, beaten to death, or even murdered.

My beautiful female do not base your relationship off of what a guy did in the past; base your relationship off of what he is doing now. If he is sweet and kind that is good, but if he is physically abusive that is bad and you should not continue to date him. You are a beautiful female who deserve to be treated with kindness and respect and not physically abused.

Whatever you do; do not stay in an abusive relationship or date an abusive guy because he has the potential to be a great guy. Just because a guy has the potential to be a great guy does not mean he will choose to be one. Everyone has the potential to be great; but if you choose not to act on it means nothing.

If you notice that the guy you are dating is becoming possessive, very jealous, and verbally abusive on a regular basis there is a very good chance that this guy can become physically abusive towards you.

Remember, you are a special gift from God and you deserve someone who will realize how special and wonderful you are.

VERBAL ABUSE

My beautiful female I want you to know that physical abuse is not the only form of abuse you may experience from an abuser. Some abusers may use verbal abuse. A person who uses verbal abuse may not leave physical scars on you, but the abuser will leave emotional scars on you.

Emotional scars can have a very negative impact on your life now and in the future. In other words; my beautiful female, you can carry around with you the negative self-image that your abuser planted in your head and in your heart now and for the rest of your life.

For those of you who do not know what verbal abuse is let me explain it to you. Verbal abuse is a use of negative words or words used negatively to destroy a person's self-esteem. The words that will be used will be used in a demeaning, insulting, degrading, humiliating, and hurtful way.

Being with a person who is verbally abusive can cause you emotional damage and harm. Listed below are some examples of verbal abuse.

1st Example – Nobody else will ever want you.

2nd Example – You are so ugly.

3rd Example – You are the ugliest girl I have ever dated.

4th Example – You will never be as good as my ex-girlfriend.

5th Example – You are so dumb.

6th Example – You can't do anything right.

7th Example – You are so fat.

8th Example – You will never be as pretty as my ex- girlfriend.

9th Example – You are so stupid.

10th Example – You would be cute if you were not so fat.

11th Example – If I did not feel sorry for you I would leave you.

12th Example – You ain't nothing but a hoe (whore).

13th Example – Look at you; you always dressing like a slut.

14th Example – Your hair is so nappy.

15th Example – Why can't you be more like your sister?

16th Example – Why you always acting like a Bitch?

17th Example – You will always be dumb and stupid.

18th Example – You ain't nothing but a slut.

19th Example – You are so skinny.

20th Example – You need to go on a diet you are getting fat.

21st Example – You are an ugly black thang.

22nd Example – You look anorexic.

23rd Example – You got an ugly smile.

24th Example – If you were not fat I would not cheat on you.

25th Example – You look like a boy with your hair short.

26th Example – If it was not for me you would be nothing.

27th Example – I am the only friend you got so you better hope I never leave you.

28th Example – Nobody wants you.

29th Example – You ain't nothing but a hoe just like your sister.

30th Example – If you were not so dumb I would not cheat on you.

31st Example – You are the dumbest girl I ever dated.

32nd Example – You are a stupid Bitch.

33rd Example – You would be cute if you were not so black.

34th Example – If you were not so ugly I would not cheat on you.

35th Example – You are the stupidest girl I ever dated.

36th Example – Nobody will ever love you.

37th Example – I see why all your boyfriends cheat on you.

38th Example – You are worthless.

39th Example – You are a dumb bitch.

40th Example – You would be pretty if you were not so skinny.
I want you to know that you should never believe anything said to you by a person who is verbally abusive. Your abuser wants to make you feel bad about yourself because he is not happy with himself. Plus, if he can get you to believe you are worthless then he knows you will never leave him. Especially, since you believe no one else will ever want you.

If you were to constantly subject yourself to the negative words from your abuser it would plant a negative seed (negative words) in your head and in your heart. Every time your abuser would say those negative words to you that negative seed that your abuser planted in your head and heart will grow. The more it grows the lower your self-esteem will become. The lower your self-esteem goes the more likely you are to stay with you abuser.

One of the goals of a guy who is verbally abusive to the female he is dating is to make her feel bad about herself so she will not leave him. A verbally abusive person needs to feel important. One ways he can do that is to make you feel bad about yourself. When you feel bad about yourself you will do just about any-thing to keep the person you are with because you feel you can-not get anyone else. That extra attention that is given to your abuser is what he needs in order to feel important.

Some abusers verbally abuse the female they are with because they feel inferior. These guys are verbally abusive because it gives them a sense of importance and power to make that female feel worthless. By making her feel worthless it takes that inferiority feeling that they once felt away from them. The only thing is that the abuser will never admit that he feels inferior when it comes to you and that is why he is verbally abusive towards you.

Also, some verbally abusive guys have realized that they can get more attention from the females they are dating by being verbally abusive. In other words, the guy who is verbally abusive is rewarded with attention for his bad behavior; verbal abuse.

If a guy's verbally abusive behavior continues to escalate it can turn into physical abuse which can lead to you having serious internal and external injuries or even death.

My beautiful female you do not deserve to be demeaned, insulted, degraded, or humiliated. You deserve to be loved, protected, cherished, and respected.

If the person you are dating is verbally abusive towards you; you should leave that person alone. Having to listen to someone constantly verbally abuse you can cause you to develop low self-esteem. You do not deserve to have to endure such hurtful and destructive behavior from a person you are dating; you deserve to be treated with kindness and respect.

LINES

My beautiful female as you go through life you will encounter guys who are only interested in having sex with you and nothing more. These guys are willing to use any and every line they can think of to convince you to have sex with them and yes they will lie if they believe it will get you to have sex with them.

In some cases the guys will try to convince you to date them believing it would be easier to convince you to have sex with if you are dating. Just so you know these guys are not trying to be your boyfriend they are only dating you so you will have sex with them.

Listed below are some of the lines guys will use to try to convince you to have sex with them as well as the lines they will use to try to convince you to date them.

Lines Guys Will Use To Try To Get You To Have Sex With Them

1st Line - This is what boyfriends and girlfriends do.

2nd Line - I love you.

3rd Line - If you was not going to give me some why you let me come over.

4th Line - This will make our relationship stronger.

5th Line - I will always love you.

6th Line - Since you're scared we do not have to do anything.

7th Line - Just let me put the tip in.

8th Line - If you won't do it someone else will.

9th Line - I knew you were not for real; you ain't nothing but a dick tease.

10th Line - If you love me you will.

11th Line - Everybody's doing it.

12th Line - You know you want it.

13th Line - If you do it I won't tell.

14th Line - If you were not going to give me some why you come over.

15th Line - If you do this I will never leave you.

16th Line - Let's just do it this time and I won't ask you no more.

17th Line – You're so beautiful.

18th Line - Just let me rub it down there I won't stick it in.

19th Line - You know I love you right? So we good?

20th Line - It won't hurt; I'll take it easy.

21st Line - You know you want this.

22nd Line - This is what people do if they really love each other.

23rd Line - You need an older man like me because I can teach you things.

24th Line - I see you ain't ready for this; you still young.

25th Line - This is how you show your boyfriend you really like him.

26th Line - I thought you said you loved me; I knew you were lying.

27th Line - If you were a real woman you would do it.

28th Line - If you do not give me some I will get blue balls.

29th Line - I thought you were ready for a real relationship; I guess I was wrong.

30th Line - SHHH don't say nothing just relax.

31st Line - You should let me hit dat (that).

32nd Line – You look like you got some good pussy; you should let me get some

33rd Line - You are so beautiful I just can't help myself.

34th Line – Sex ain't a sin if you do it with the person you love.

35th Line – God created sex for people who love each other and we love each other.

36th Line – You know you want this big dick.

37th Line – You won't get pregnant if it is your first time.

38th Line – It is my first time too.

39th Line – I am going to stop coming over to see you since you will not give me some.

40th Line – I have been dating you for a while; how much longer do I have to wait?

41st Line – I want to make your first time special.

42nd Line – You should let me be your first because I won't hurt you.

43rd Line – I am a virgin and I want you to be my first.

44th Line – You look so good; I don't want anybody else to have you.

45th Line – My girlfriend said she wants to wait until she is married and I got needs.

46th Line – Let me use my finger that way you can still be a virgin.

47th Line – Can I go down on you?

48th Line – Let's get a room; we don't have to do nothing if you don't want to.

49th Line – Ain't nothing wrong with kissing.

50th Line – Just five minutes and I promise I will stop asking.

51st Line - I never felt this way about a girl before.

52nd Line – Girl, you got my dick so hard you should just give me some

53rd Line – You da girl I am going to marry so it is ok for you to have sex with me.

54th Line – No one makes me feel like you do.

55th Line – Lets skip school and get a room.

56th Line – Baby you know you are all I ever wanted.

57th Line – You should let me go down on you.

My beautiful female your body is a rare and precious jewel and being the owner of that precious treasure you need to be extremely selective of who gets to have your rare and precious jewel. Something as valuable as your body should not be passed around as if it is a raggedy dirty old shoe; something worthless, i should be cherished. My beautiful female you should never treat your body as if it is community property because it is not. Remember, your body is a rare and precious jewel and a rare and precious jewel should be cherished and protected from harm and danger by you at all times. Having sex with a guy just because he want to have sex with you is not how you cherish and protect your rare and precious jewel.

Lines Older Guys Will Use To Try To Get You To Date Them

1st Line – You are very mature for your age.

2nd Line – You need an older guy like me because I can teach you things.

3rd Line – Older women have too many issues (problems); that is why I need someone young like you.

4th Line – We can just be friends.

5th Line – You are not like other girls your age you are more mature.

6th Line – You are so beautiful.

7th Line – You and I could be good together.

8th Line – I wish I had someone in my life like you.

9th Line – I like talking to you because you understand me.

10th Line – If I can find a girl like you to date I would be straight.

11th Line – Older women do not know how to have fun; that is why I need someone young like you.

12th Line – I just want to take care of you.

13th Line – If you were my woman I would take really good care of you.

14th Line – I wish I had somebody in my life like you because I would spend all my money on her.

15th Line – If you were my woman I would give you whatever you want.

16th Line - You need an older guy like me because these young guys do not know how to treat you like a woman.

17th Line – I feel like I have known you all my life.

18th Line - Older women do not know how to appreciate a good man.

19th Line – Older women are too bossy that is why I need someone young like you.

20th Line – Age ain't nothing but a number.

21st Line – You need an older guy like me because I can do things for you that these young guys can't do.

22nd Line – There is something about you that I just can't resist.

23rd Line – Girls your age are usually not this mature. You and I should go out sometimes.

24th Line – You so pretty; I just want to spend some time with you.

25th Line – I usually do not talk to girls your age, but you seem very mature.

My beautiful female do not fall for the lines older guys will use on you. These older men are only trying to date you so they can convince you to have sex with them. Do not allow them to abuse your body sexually. Your body is a rare and precious jewel and a rare and precious jewel should be cherished and protected. Having sex with these older men is not how you cherish and protect your rare and precious jewel. Plus, you should only give your rare and precious jewel to the person that loves, cherish, respect, honor, and protects you. Older men who prey on females do not love, cherish, respect, honor, or protect them. Therefore; they should not give them your rare and precious jewel.

Lines Married Men Will Use To Try To Get You To Date Them

1st Line – My wife just do not understand me like you do.

2nd Line – My wife ain't affectionate and I can tell you would be.

3rd Line – I am about to get a divorce.

4th Line – Me and my wife ain't really married we just live together for the sake of the kids.

5th Line – Me and my wife have an open marriage.

6th Line – Me and my wife just do not get along like we do.

7th Line – My wife do not love me no more.

8th Line – I have not had sex with my wife in over a year.

9th Line – Me and my wife are separated.

10th Line - I just wear a ring I am not really married.

11th Line – Me and my wife have grown apart.

12th Line – You and I have so much in common unlike me and my wife.

13th Line – There is something about you that I just cannot resist.

14th Line – I am so lonely.

15th Line – My wife cheated on me.

16th Line – We are friends and friends can hang out with one another.

17th Line – My wife stays with me because she ain't got nowhere else to go.

18th Line – Me and my wife are like roommates; we are not a couple.

19th Line – My wife do not care if I date other people.

20th Line – I am leaving my wife.

21st Line – It is over between me and my wife.

22nd Line – My wife do not like to do the things I like to do, but you do.

23rd Line – You are my soul mate

24th Line – I do not love my wife anymore; I love you.

My beautiful female you need to beware of married men who try to date females while they are married. These men are only interested in dating you purely for sexual reasons. In other words they do not want to be with you; they only want to have sex with you. You must know that despite what these married men have said to you they are not going to leave their wife to be with you. Everything they told you was a lie. They only told you those things so it will be easier to convince you to have sex with them. Do not let a married man abuse your body sexually. Remember, your body is a rare and precious jewel and a rare and precious jewel is meant to be cherished and protected from harm and danger by you at all times. Having sex with a married man is not how you cherish and protect your rare and precious jewel. Plus, you should only give your rare and precious jewel to the person that loves, cherish, respect, honor, and protects you. Any married man who is willing to cheat on his wife does not respect his wife or you; nor does he respect females in general. Therefore; married men should not be given your rare and precious jewel.

SEXTING

My beautiful female you may feel that there is nothing wrong with Sexting. No one forced you to take a naked picture or a partially naked picture of yourself. No one forced you to text your partially naked picture or your fully naked picture to a guy or several guys. Well, my beautiful female Sexting can lead to you experiencing several undesirable things. Listed below are some of the undesirable things you may have to endure because you chose to text a partially naked or a fully naked picture of yourself to a guy or some guys.

Undesirable Things

1st Undesirable Thing

Someone can post your partially naked picture or your fully naked picture on social media; which means anybody and everybody can see it. I want you to know once your partially naked picture or your fully naked picture is in cyber space it is there forever.

2nd Undesirable Thing

Your partially naked picture or your fully naked picture could be texted to all the people in your school. This can lead to a lot of people talking about you and calling you very horrible names. Plus, those people can take that picture of you and text it to other people and those people can take your picture and text it to other people. Now people in different schools will be looking at your partially naked picture or your fully naked picture.

3rd Undesirable Thing

You may be charged with distributing child pornography; all because you texted a partially naked picture or a fully naked picture of a minor even though the minor is you. If you are found guilty of distributing child pornography you can spend time in jail. You will have to register yourself as a sex offender. Now that you are a registered sex offender you will not be able to be around minor children or live with minor children. If you have younger brothers and sisters you will have to live somewhere else. Or your brothers and sisters will have to leave their home and live somewhere else. Plus, you will not be allowed to live 500 to 1000 feet from parks, play grounds, or schools. In other words you cannot live anywhere where there will be minor children around.

4th Undesirable Thing

You will have a difficult time trying to find a job in the future because you have been convicted of a felony (child pornography). Just so you know a lot of businesses do not hire people with felonies.

5th Undesirable Thing

You may have a difficult time finding a job because your future employers may have seen your partially naked picture or your fully naked picture and decides not to hire you because your behavior compromises the integrity of their company.

My precious female you need to know that just because someone ask you to send them a partially naked picture or a fully naked picture of you does not mean you have to give that person one. Just because a guy wants to see your body does not mean he deserve to see it. Your body is a rare and precious jewel and a rare and precious jewel is meant to be cherished and protected by you at all times. Sending partially naked pictures or fully naked pictures of your body to every guy who wants to see it is not an act of cherishing and protecting your rare and precious jewel.

SEXUALLY TRANSMITTED DISEASES

Sexually Transmitted Disease: Any disease that is transmitted through sexual contact. These diseases are caused by micro-organisms that survive on the skin or the mucus membranes of the genital area. These microorganisms are transmitted via semen, vaginal secretions, or blood during Sex acts and sexual intercourse. Because the genital areas provide moisture and warmth it makes for the perfect environment for the proliferation of bacteria, viruses, and yeasts.

My beautiful female for those of you who are sexually active I need you to realize that you must be extremely careful when engaging in sexual intercourse and oral sex. Engaging in this activity irresponsibly can lead to you developing a Sexually Transmitted Disease (STD).

Just so you know some Sexually Transmitted Diseases are curable if detected in its early stages. Others are not curable no matter when you detect them. Also, some Sexually Transmitted Diseases can develop into new and worse diseases if not treated immediately. Some STDs can cause people to take medication for the rest of their lives. Also, some females have become infertile because of the STD they have contracted.

My beautiful female you should know that you can have a Sexually Transmitted Disease for months and not know you have one simply because of the way a female's body is designed.

When a female has a Sexually Transmitted Disease it is usually inside the vagina where she cannot see it. Therefore; she will not the visit a gynochologist annually for check-ups.

When you are infected with a STD you can experience signs and symptoms from the STD that you have. Listed below are some of the symptoms you may experience when a STD is present.

- Abnormal discharge
- Stinging when urinating
- Discharge having a fishy odor
- Fever
- Pain when urinating
- Nausea
- Lower abdominal pain
- Intense itching
- Pelvic pain
- Burning when urination
- Swollen vagina
- Blood in your vaginal discharge
- Aching body
- Bleeding between menstrual cycle
- Hair loss
- Pearl colored bumps with indented core in the middle
- Vomiting
- Diarrhea
- Jaundice
- Itchy skin
- Joint pain
- Fatigue
- Having blue, yellow, or green discharge
- Itching around sex organs
- Discomfort
- Difficulty urinating
- Abdominal pain
- Irregular menstrual bleeding
- Pain during sexual intercourse
- Low immune system

- Damage to your fallopian tubes
- Damage to your uterus
- Chills
- Cramps throughout the months
- Constipation
- Damage to your ovaries
- Painful fluid filled bumps inside the vagina
- Painful fluid filled bumps on your cervix
- Irritated vagina
- Sores, bumps, puss filled bumps on the small and large lips on the vagina
- Sores, bumps, puss filled bumps around your vagina
- Sores, bumps, puss filled bumps around your anus
- Sores
- Swollen lymph glands
- Skin growths in clusters
- Fluid filled Bubo
- Tender lymph nodes in the groin area
- Grayish colored bump around genital area
- Itchy bumps
- Small red bumps around the genital area
- Small red bumps around the breast
- Inflammation of the lymph nodes
- Flesh tone colored bumps around the inner thigh
- Flesh tone colored bumps around the genital area

If a female has a Sexually Transmitted Disease and she does not seek treatment for it; it can lead to other health issue. Some of the other health issues a female can experience from an untreated Sexually Transmitted Disease are

- Pelvic Inflammatory Disease (PID)
- Sever pelvic pain
- Damage to your fallopian tubes
- Damage to your uterus
- Ectopic pregnancy (your baby grow outside your uterus).

HOW TO STAY SAFE IF YOU ARE SEXUALLY ACTIVE

My beautiful female if you are sexually active I would prefer you stop engaging in this activity and wait until you are ready to handle everything that comes with being sexually active. If you are not going to stop having sex listed below are some tips you can follow to help keep yourself safe while you are sexually active.

Safety Tips

1st Safety Tip – Always look at the guy's penis
before you have sex with him.

By looking at the guy's penis you will be able to see if he has a Sexually Transmitted Disease present. If the guy has a Sexually Transmitted Disease there will be visible signs you can see. Listed below are the visible signs to look for are:

- Sores, bumps, lesions, or puss filled bumps on the head of the penis
- Sores, bumps, lesions, or puss filled bumps on the shaft of the penis
- Discharge from the penis (fluids dripping from the head of the penis)
- Swollen sacks (testicles, balls)
- Sores, bumps, lesions, or puss filled bumps around the anus
- Sores, bumps, lesions, or puss filled bumps around the inner

thighs

- Sores, bumps, lesions, or puss filled bumps around the genital area

Other things that can indicate that a guy is infected with a STD are:

- Difficulty urinating

- Intense itching

If you notice that the guy is infected with a Sexually Transmitted Disease I strongly recommend that you do not engage in any sex activity with him. If you decide to have sex with him anyway you will get the same Sexually Transmitted Disease that he has.

If you are too scared to look at the guy's penis then you are not ready to have sex; simply because you will not do everything necessary to protect your rare and precious jewel from harm and danger.

2nd Safety Tip – Always use a condom when having sex.

If the semen is infected with a Sexually Transmitted Disease (STD) it will not come in contact with your vagina because it is inside the condom. If the guy has any sores, bumps, lesions, or puss filled bumps on the head of his penis it will not come in contact with your vagina because the condom is covering it up. My precious female you need to know that condoms only work when they do not come off, break, have a hole in it, or if they are old. If any of those things were to happen to the condom you will become infected with the same Sexually Transmitted Disease the guy has. Plus, if the guy has any sores, bumps, lesions, or puss filled bumps on the shaft of his penis near his pubic hair the condom will not cover it which means you will become infected with that Sexually Transmitted Disease too.

If you have sex with a guy and he has a STD and he did not use a condom you will get infected with the same sexually transmitted disease that he has. Some of the STDs you can get from having sex without using a condom is:

- Human Immunodeficiency Virus - HIV which eventually turns

into Acquired Immune Deficiency Syndrome AIDS
- Herpes
- Syphilis
- Gonorrhea
- Chlamydia
- Genital Warts
- Trichomonas
- Hepatitis
- Lymphogranuloma Venereum
- Chacroid
- Cytomegalovirus (CMV)
- Molluscum Contagiosum
- Scabies

Some of the symptoms you can experience if you were to contract one of these Sexually Transmitted Diseases are:
- Abnormal discharge
- Stinging when urinating
- Discharge having a fishy odor
- Fever
- Pain when urinating
- Nausea
- Lower abdominal pain
- Intense itching
- Pelvic pain
- Burning when urination
- Swollen vagina
- Blood in your vaginal discharge
- Aching body
- Bleeding between menstrual cycle
- Hair loss
- Pearl colored bumps with indented core in the middle
- Vomiting
- Diarrhea
- Jaundice
- Itchy skin
- Joint pain

- Fatigue
- Having blue, yellow, or green discharge
- Itching around sex organs
- Discomfort
- Difficulty urinating
- Abdominal pain
- Irregular menstrual bleeding
- Pain during sexual intercourse
- Low immune system
- Damage to your fallopian tubes
- Damage to your uterus
- Chills
- Cramps throughout the months
- Constipation
- Damage to your ovaries
- Painful fluid filled bumps inside the vagina
- Painful fluid filled bumps on your cervix
- Irritated vagina
- Sores, bumps, puss filled bumps on the small and large lips on the vagina
- Sores, bumps, puss filled bumps around your vagina
- Sores, bumps, puss filled bumps around your anus
- Sores
- Swollen lymph glands
- Skin growths in clusters
- Fluid filled Bubo
- Tender lymph nodes in the groin area
- Grayish colored bump around genital area
- Itchy bumps
- Small red bumps around the genital area
- Small red bumps around the breast
- Inflammation of the lymph nodes
- Flesh tone colored bumps around the inner thigh
- Flesh tone colored bumps around the genital area

My precious female if you were to get Chlamydia or Gonorrhea and you do not seek treatment it will turn into a new disease

called *Pelvic Inflammatory Disease* (PID). Some of the symptoms you will experience from Pelvic Inflammatory Disease are:
- Yellow or green vaginal discharge
- Discharge with a foul odor
- Irregular menstrual bleeding
- Pain when urinating
- Abdominal pain
-Vomiting
- Diarrhea
- Longer periods
- Pelvic pain
- Cramps throughout the month
- Pain in lower back
- Pain in the rectum
- Fatigue
- Fever
- Chills
- Dull pain in stomach
- Ectopic pregnancy (baby growing outside the uterus)
- Pain in the anus
- Pain when having sexual intercourse
- Sores, bumps, puss filled bumps on and around your inner thigh

My beautiful female if you have Pelvic Inflammatory Disease you will have it occur in:
- The fallopian tubes
- The lining of the uterus
- The upper genital tract
- The uterus
- The ovaries
- Throughout the pelvic area

My lovely female if you decide to have sex with a guy who has Pubic Lice you will get Pubic Lice too; even if he uses a condom. When you get Pubic Lice from having sexual intercourse you will have them in your pubic hair. You should also know that Pubic Lice will lay 2-3 eggs daily and continue to multiply until you use medication to get rid of them. This parasite will bite you while they feed on your blood and defecated in your pubic hair until you use medication to get rid of them. The only way to not get Pubic Lice is to not engage in vaginal, anal, or oral sex. My beautiful female if you realize the guy you were going to have sex with has a sexually transmitted disease I recommend that you do not have sex with him. Even if he states he will wear a condom you should still tell him no. Just so you know if that condom was to break, come off, or have a whole in it you will become infected with that STD he has. Never put your life in jeopardy for sex. Better safe than sorry.

3rd Safety Tip – Select a gynecologist.

My beautiful female because you are sexually active you will need to start having annual checkups (Pap smear) as well as get tested for Sexually Transmitted Diseases (STDs). Having a healthy cervix can help prevent bacteria from the vagina from spreading to your reproductive organs. If you have an untreated STD it can cause the cervix to become infected. If the cervix is infected it will be unable to protect your reproductive organs which can lead to you experiencing infertility, Pelvic Inflammatory Disease, Ectopic Pregnancy, and pelvic pain. That is why it is important to get test for STDs if you are sexually active.

By having your own gynecologist you will have a gynecologist who is familiar with your medical history. Plus, he or she will be familiar with your body and will be able to tell if you are infected with a STD or if your body is just designed that way.

My precious female; the only way to prevent yourself from contracting a Sexually Transmitted Disease is to not have sex; vaginal, anal, or oral. If you are going to have sex please do everything you possibly can do to not get infected with a Sexually Transmitted Disease.

PREGNANCY

My beautiful female I want you to know that every time you have sex there is a chance that you may become pregnant. If you do not want to become pregnant there is only one thing you can do to guarantee that you never become pregnant and that is not to have sex. If you are not going to stop having sex and you do not want to get pregnant it is up to you to do everything you can to prevent that from happening. Listed below there are several things you can do to help prevent yourself from becoming pregnant.

Things you can do to avoid becoming pregnant

1st Thing – select a gynecologist.

By having a gynecologist; he or she can help you to select which birth control would be best for you. Also, your gynecologist can go over the different side effect you may experience. You should know that there is still a chance that you may become pregnant while using birth control.

2nd Thing – Always use condoms every time you have sex.

By using condoms you will not become pregnant when the guy ejaculates inside you. You should know that condoms do not work when they come off, have a hole in it, if they break, or if they are old. If any of these things were to happen to the condom sperm will enter into your vagina and you can become pregnant.

My beautiful female if you ever become pregnant you will need to be brave and tell your parents and the father of the child.

That way they can help you make the decision that is best for you; whether that is keeping your baby, giving your baby up for adoption, or even having an abortion. I know this is a very scary time for you, but you are a strong and courageous female and you can tell your parents and the father of the child that you are pregnant.

If you are considering hiding your pregnancy and getting rid of the baby once he or she is born I suggest you do not do that. If you abandon you child after you have given birth you can be charged with child endangerment and neglect which means you can go to jail. If you cause your baby to die after you have given birth you can be charged with murder or man slaughter which mean you can go to jail. The best thing for you to do is tell your parents and the father of the child you are pregnant so they can help you to do what is best for you and the baby.

If you are thinking that getting an abortion every time you get pregnant is an effective means of birth control you are absolutely wrong. Having multiple abortions can make it difficult for you to carry a baby when you do decide to become a mommy.

ORAL SEX

My beautiful female, there are a lot of females engaging in oral sex with guys and some are engaging in oral sex with guys and females. A lot of guys and females will try to pressure you into participating in this sex act with them. They will tell you that it is safe, you will still be a virgin, you will not get pregnant, and you cannot get a Sexually Transmitted Disease. My precious female these individuals told you all these things in hopes of you giving into the peer pressure of performing oral sex on him or her or for you to let him or her perform oral sex on you.

What you need to know is that some of what they told is true. For instance: you will not get pregnant. You will still be a virgin, but only in relation to intercourse (penetration) as far as sex acts you will not be a virgin. As for oral sex being safe sex and you cannot get a STD that is absolutely WRONG. Oral sex is NOT safe sex and you CAN get a Sexually Transmitted Disease.

Your Mouth Becoming Infected With A Sexually Transmitted Disease

If you were to perform oral sex on a male or a female and that person was infected with a Sexually Transmitted Disease you will get it too. The worst part about contracting a Sexually Transmitted Disease from performing oral sex on someone is that you will have that Sexually Transmitted Disease in your mouth and throat.

My beautiful female the Sexually Transmitted Diseases you can get in your mouth and throat from performing oral sex on a guy

or a female are:
- Herpes
- Syphilis
- Gonorrhea
- Warts

Some of the symptoms you will experience from each of these Sexually Transmitted Diseases are listed below.

Herpes (Herpes Simplex Virus I)

- Small red blisters on and around your mouth as well as in your throat
- Reoccurring out breaks on and in your mouth as well as in your throat
- Fever
- Difficulty swallowing
- A sore throat
- Swollen glands in your neck
- Fluid filled blisters on your throat
- Fluid filled blisters in and around your mouth
- Pain
- Discomfort

Syphilis
- Mucus patches in your mouth
- Mucus patches on your throat
- Ulcers in your mouth
- Ulcers in throat.
- Difficulty swallowing
- Inflammatory lesion in your mouth
- Inflammatory lesion on your throat
- Swollen glands in your throat.
- Pain
- Discomfort
- A sore throat

Gonorrhea

- A sore throat
- Difficulty swallowing
- Discomfort

- Puss like substance on your tonsils
- Puss like substance on the back of your throat
- Inflamed tonsils
- Inflamed throat
- Pain.

Warts

- Difficulty swallowing
- Discomfort
- A sore throat
- Pain
- Warts inside your mouth
- Warts in your throat

My beautiful female you should know that there is another Sexually Transmitted Disease you can get if you perform oral sex on a guy or a female. That Sexually Transmitted Disease is called *Pubic Lice* also known as "crabs".

Pubic Lice

If you were to get Pubic Lice you will not have them in your mouth and throat you will have them on your scalp and you will have them in the hair on your face. You will have Pubic Lice in your eyelashes, your eyebrows, and any other fine traces of hair you may have on your face. If you have any traces of hair on your arms there is a very good chance that you will have Pubic Lice there too.

You will also have intense itching because the Pubic Lice are biting you while they are feeding on your blood and defecating on your scalp and face. The Pubic Lice that you have on your scalp and face will continue to multiply by laying 2-3 eggs every day until you use medication to get rid of them and their eggs.

As you can see performing oral sex on a guy or a female is not as safe as you thought it was.

You must remember that your body is a rare and precious jewel and a rare and precious jewel is meant to be cherished and protected from harm and danger by you at all times by you.

Your Vagina Becoming Infected With
A Sexually Transmitted Disease

My precious female if you decide to let a guy or a female perform oral sex on you and their mouth and throat is infected with a Sexually Transmitted Disease that Sexually Transmitted Disease will spread to your vagina. The Sexually Transmitted Diseases that can spread from someone's mouth and throat to a female's vagina are:
- Herpes
- Syphilis
- Gonorrhea
- Warts

Listed below are some of the symptoms you will experience if your vagina becomes infected with a Sexually Transmitted Disease because the person who performed oral sex on you had a mouth and throat that was infected.

Genital Herpes (Herpes Simplex Virus 2)

If Herpes were to spread to your vagina because the person who performed oral sex on you had a mouth and throat that was infected with the Herpes Virus 1 you will have these symptoms.
- Itching in the vagina
- Itching in the rectum
- Itching in the anus
- Burning in the vagina
- Burning in the rectum
- Burning in the anus
- Tenderness in the groin area
- Swelling in the groin area
- Fever
- Fatigue
- Loss of appetite
- Irritability
- Flu-like symptoms
- Painful blisters

- Fluid fill blister inside your vagina
- Fluid fill blister on your cervix
- Fluid fill blister on your labia (vagina lips)
- Reoccurring out breaks
- Extreme pain
- Discomfort

Just so you know Genital Herpes is extremely contagious and once you have it you will have it for life.

Syphilis

If you were to receive oral sex from a person whose mouth and throat was infected with the Syphilis Virus your vagina will become infected with the Syphilis virus. Once your vagina is infected with the Syphilis Virus you will go through four different stages of Syphilis: _Primary Stage, Secondary Stage, Latent Stage,_ and _Tertiary Stage._ Listed below are the symptoms you will experience from each stage of the Syphilis Virus.

Primary Stage

The symptom you will have in the _Primary Stage_ is:
- Developing Chancre sores

Secondary Stage

Symptoms you will have in the _Secondary Stage_ are:
- Aching body
- Fever
- Hair loss
- Nausea
- Sore throat
- Swollen glands
- Fatigue
- Broad based papules (lumps and warts)
- Headaches
- Malaise (vague depression)

Latent Stage

During the _Latent Stage_ of the Syphilis Virus you will not experience any symptoms. It will give you the impression that you are no longer infected with the Syphilis Virus, but that is not true. You are still infected with the Syphilis Virus. Syphilis in the Latent Stage can remain latent (hidden) for many years. If the Syphilis Virus has not been treated by the third stage (Latent Stage) you will move on to the last stage of the Syphilis Virus which is the *Tertiary Stage*.

Tertiary Stage

 Once you have moved to the *Tertiary Stage* your body has totally become infected with the *Spirochetes Bacteria*. Now that your entire body is infected with the *Spirochetes Bacteria* it can cause problems with the:

- Eyes
- Heart
- Brain
- Nervous system
- Joints
- Spinal cord (neurosyphilis)
- Heart and blood vessels
- Nervous system

You will also experience inflammatory lesions on the:

- Bones
- Skin
- Cardiovascular system
- Reproductive organs
- Upper and lower respiratory tract
- Abdominal organs
- Eyes
- Mouth
- Lymph nodes

Once you develop Cardiovascular Syphilis this can cause complication such as:

- Blindness
- Heart diseases
- Mental illness (insanity)

My lovely female you can also develop neurological problems from having the Syphilis Virus. Plus, you can die from having the Syphilis Virus.

Gonorrhea

If Gonorrhea was to spread to your vagina because the person who perform oral sex on you had a mouth and throat that was infected with Gonorrhea you will experience these symptoms:
- Yellow or green vaginal discharge
- Vaginal bleeding between menstrual cycles
- Burning when urinating
- Pain when urinating
- Chronic abdominal pain
- Rectal infection
If you were to develop a rectal infection you can experience:
- Discharge from the rectum
- Anal itching
- Soreness
- Bleeding from rectum
- Painful bowel movements
My precious female if Gonorrhea goes untreated it will lead to more complication with the body; some of those complications are:
- Infertility (unable to have children)
- Ectopic pregnancy (baby growing outside of the womb – usually in the fallopian tubes)
- Damage to the fallopian tubes
- Pelvic Inflammatory Disease (PID)
If you were to develop *Pelvic Inflammatory Disease* because you did not seek treatment for the Gonorrhea you had you will experience:
- Internal abscesses (puss-filled pockets)
- Chronic pelvic pain
- Damage to the fallopian tubes which can cause infertility
- Damage to your uterus
- Damage to your ovaries
- Damage to the tissue in and near the uterus and ovaries
- Increase risk of developing ectopic pregnancy
- Unusual vaginal discharge (yellow or green in color)
- Discharge with a foul odor
- Pain when urinating

- Pain when having sexual intercourse
- Abdominal pain
- Pain in the lower abdominal area
- Fever
- Chills
- Nausea
- Vomiting
- Irregular menstrual bleeding
- Fatigue
- Diarrhea
- Right upper abdominal pain
- Pain in lower back
- Pain in the rectum
- Pain in the anus
- Pelvic pain
- Dull pain in the stomach
- Tenderness in the stomach
- Longer periods
- Scarring
- Ectopic pregnancy
- Spotting throughout the month
- Cramps throughout the month

Genital Warts

My beautiful female if Warts were to spread to your vagina because the person who perform oral sex on you had a mouth and throat that was infected with Warts you will experience:
- Itching around sex organs
- Burning around sex organs
- Painless growths located on damp or moist surfaces in and on your vagina
- Tiny, soft, pinkish, or reddish spots
- Bleeding
- Difficulty urinating
- Discomfort
- Unusual colored vaginal discharge
- White/yellowish/gray bumpy warts on the vagina

- White/yellowish/gray bumpy warts on the anus
- Cauliflower-like irregular shape growths

My beautiful female you should know that there is another Sexually Transmitted Disease you can get if you allow a guy or a female to perform oral sex on you. That Sexually Transmitted Disease is *Pubic Lice* also known as "crabs".

Pubic Lice

If the person who is performing oral sex on you is infected with Pubic Lice in their eyelashes, their eye brows, and on their scalp you will become infected with Pubic Lice too. You will not have them inside your vagina you will have Pubic Lice in your pubic mound; in pubic hair.

Once you are infected with Pubic Lice you will have intense itching on your pubic mound. You will be itching because the Pubic Lice are biting you while they are feeding on your blood and defecating in your pubic hair. If the Pubic Lice are not treated immediately they will begin to lay eggs. The Pubic lice will lay 2-3 eggs call Nits, daily. Those eggs are attached to the hair shaft on the genitals (penis and vagina). The eggs usually hatches within 6-10 days and produce baby Pubic Lice call *Nymphs.* Within 15 days the Nymphs will grow into adult lice and multiply again. Both Nymphs and adult Pubic lice feed on your blood.

Just so you know if anyone was to sleep in your bed once you are infected with the parasite they will become infected too. They will become infected because the Pubic Lice are on your sheets and bed spread waiting to attach itself to the hair on someone's body.

When you find out that you are infected with Pubic Lice make sure you wash all the linen on your bed. Plus, make sure you wash all of the clothes that you have worn and all the towels and wash cloths you have used. This need to be done immediately to make sure you have killed all the parasites and their eggs that was on you bedding, towels, wash cloths, and cloths.

As you can see allowing a guy or a female to perform oral sex on

you is not as safe as you thought it was.
My beautiful female you must remember that your body is a rare and precious jewel and a rare and precious jewel is meant to be cherished and protected from harm and danger by you at all times. By allowing a guy or a female to perform oral sex on you may cause your rare and precious jewel harm and damage. Also, you can cause your body harm and damage to your rare and precious jewel by performing oral sex on a guy or a female whose genital (penis or vagina) is infected with a Sexually Transmitted Disease.

INTERNET SAFETY

My beautiful female we use the internet to do many different things. We use the internet to watch movies, play games, watch music videos, chat with people in various locations, and to shop. What you need to realize is that not all people use the internet for entertainment. There are people who use the internet to steal people's identity and to steal people's money. Some people use the internet to set up meeting locations in order to rape and robbed people. Also, there are some people who use the internet to set up meetings and dates to have sex with under age female. My beautiful female I want you to know that there are several things you can do to stay safe while using the internet.

Safety Tips

1st Safety Tip – Never listed your full name, date of birth, complete mailing address, and social security number on any social networking websites.
If you were to list all those things someone will be able to steal your identity. Once someone steals your identity you can be held accountable for a lot of debt that you did not make. They can also have you linked to a criminal act which can lead to you going to jail for something you did not do.

2nd Safety Tip – When shopping on line use a prepaid debit card when paying for your purchases.
By using a prepaid Credit Card your checking account information will not be stolen if someone hacks into that company's computer system where you made your online purchases from.

3rd Safety Tip – When shopping via the internet
be sure that you are on a secure website.
If you are not sure if a website is secure look for the pad lock
icon at the bottom of the page; sometimes the pad lock icon is
located in the address bar

Things A Social Media Predator
Would Type Or Say

My beautiful female social media is a very good way to keep in touch with friends and family, but it is also used for other purposes. There are people who use social media to prey on beautiful females and even males. These individuals who prey on females via social media are grown men. These predators will chat with females via social media, skyp. face time, or a web cam with the hopes of convincing her to meet with them.

If you were to meet with a predator it can lead to you experiencing undesirable consequences. Some of the things you can experience by meeting with a predator are: being raped, getting beaten, being forced into prostitution, sold to other predators, or even murdered.

My precious female you need to understand that these predators would say whatever they think they need to say to get you to meet with them. If you are wondering would they lie to you to get you to meet with them the answer is yes; they would. Also, they would promise to give you whatever you want to get you to meet with them. Even though they know they are not going to get you all the things you asked for.

Listed below are some of the ways to tell if you are chatting with a predator.

1st Way – A predator will stress he is looking for a young female (pre-teen or teenage girl) to chat with.

2nd Way – A predator will want to know if you are a virgin or not a virgin.

3rd Way – A predator will want to meet with you in secrecy.

4th Way – A predator will be a grown man trying to talk to a pre-teen or a teenage girl.

5th Way – A predator will try to set up a meeting for sex.

6th Way - A predator will offer to buy you things in order to have sex with you.

7th Way – A predator will try to convince you that he really cares about you and that is why you should meet with him.

8th Way – A predator will offer to give you money in order to have sex with you.

9th Way – A predator will try to convince you that your parents will not understand about your relationship so do not tell them about you and him. Plus, they will tell you do not tell your parents the date, time, and place where you are going to meet each other because your parents will not let you go.

10th Way – A predator will offer to bring you drugs and alcohol to get you to have sex with him.

11th Way – A predator will want to know if you are a cop acting like a pre-teen or a teenage girl for an undercover sting operation.

12th Way – A predator will want to talk about sex and sexual things with you.

13th Way – A predator will say and promise to do anything if he believes it will convince you to meet with him.

14th Way – A predator will try to get you to do sexual thing on your web cam so he can watch.

15th Way – A predator will tell you he loves you if he feels it will get you to meet with him.

16th Way – A predator will offer to take care of you in order to get you to meet with him.

17th Way – A predator will try to get you to send him provocative or nude photos.

18th Way – A predator will offer to masturbate on his web cam so you can watch.

19th Way – A predator would try to convince you to masturbate on your webcam so he can watch you.

20th Way – A predator will say you are friends and you should meet; even though you barely know each other.

21st Way – A predator will try to make you believe you are very special that is why he chose to chat with you.

My beautiful female you must understand that these grown men are predators as well as very good liars. They know what to say to get you to believe the lies they are telling you. These predators will not stop feeding you lies until they get what they want which is for you to meet with them so they can have sex with you.

You must remember your body is a rare and precious jewel and a rare and precious jewel is meant to be cherished and protected from harm and danger by you at all times. Having sex with a predator is not an act of cherishing and protecting your rare and precious jewel. Plus, the person you have a sexual relationship with should love, cherish, honor, respect, and protect you. Social media predators do not love, cherish, honor, respect, or protect the females they manipulate; they use and abuse them. My beautiful female; if you are chatting with anyone on line do not give out any personal information about yourself. Also, do not send provocative or nude pictures to people you meet on social media; that person may be a predator. Sending predators very provocative or nude pictures of you or giving them personal information can be very dangerous. Listed below are some of the things you should never tell people you meet via social media.

1st Thing – Never tell a person you have met via social media your address because he may be a predator. This person may come to your house unannounced and cause you and your family harm.

2nd Thing – Never tell a person you have met via social media the time your parents will not be home. This person may try to come over when no one is there to protect you.

3rd Thing – Never tell a person you have met via social media your sexual status. This person may try to convince you to have sex with him by offering to buy you things, bring you drugs and alcohol, or give you money to have sex with him. If this person finds out that you are not a virgin he will try to entice you with sex. If that does not work he will offer to give you money, drugs, alcohol, and to buy you things.

4th Thing – Never tell a person you have met via social media how angry you are at your parents. If he is a predator he will try to convince you that he can and will treat you better than your parents do.

5th Thing – Never tell a person you have met via social media what school you attend. This person may come to your school looking for you. If he finds you there is a chance that he may abduct you, rape you, or physically harm you.

6th Thing – Never send provocative or nude pictures of yourself to a person you have met via social medial. This person can use your pictures to recognize you without you knowing who he is. Plus, there is a chance that he may abduct you, rape you, force you into prostitution, or even sell you to other predators who preys on young girls too. All these things can take place because he recognizes you from the picture(s) you sent him. Also, this person may trade your pictures with other people who seek out pictures of young females. Once those pictures are out in cyber space they are out there forever. Which mean any and everybody will be able to view those pictures.

My beautiful female you should know that these social media predators are very good at manipulating young female to get what they want. That is why it is very important that you know what an internet predator will type and say.

Another thing you should know about these social media predators is that sometimes they would send you very explicit videos. Those video will show the predator exposing his genitalia. In some case the video will show the predator masturbating. If you ever receive one of these videos do not delete it. Show the video to your parents so they can contact the sexual predator task force in your state.

If ever you feel you are chatting with a predator stop chatting with him and inform your parents so they can inform the proper authorities. Just so you know females can be predators too.

STRANGERS

My beautiful female you should beware of people you do not know. There are strangers who will prey on trusting beautiful females like yourself. These strangers will use your kindness as a weapon against you. It is up to you to do whatever you can to keep yourself safe when dealing with strangers. List below are some things you can do to stay safe when dealing with strangers.

Safety Tips

1st Safety Tip – Never approach a stranger's car to give him or her directions.

If you were to approach a stranger's car he can pull you into his car so he can rob you, rape you, beat you, abduct you, or murder you. In some cases the stranger will do all five things to their victims. My beautiful female it does not matter if there is a female in the car do not approach that car.

If a stranger asks you for directions you can tell him the directions from where you are standing. Do not approach a stranger's car. If a stranger cannot hear you he can go to a gas station and get directions. He can buy a navigation system for his car. He can even use the GPS feature on his cell phone. It is not your responsibility to give strangers directions because they say they are lost; what you are responsible for is keeping yourself safe at all times.

2nd Safety Tip – Never approach a stranger's car to take a flyer.

If you were to approach a stranger's car to take a flyer that stranger can pull you into his car so he could rape you, beat you, rob you, abduct you, force you into prostitution, murder you, or do all six things to you.

3rd Safety Tip - Never go with a stranger to help
him or her look for their lost pet.
My lovely female this is a line predators use all the time to get females and even boys to go with them. Some of these predators use this line to lure children away so they can abduct them, rape them, beat them, sell them to other predators, force them in to prostitution, and even murder them. That is why you should never go with a stranger to help him or her look for their lost pet. Plus, by you being a child or an adolescent the adult stranger should not be asking you to help him or her look for their pet anyway.

4th Safety Tip – Never go with a stranger who says your
parents told him (or her) to come and get you.
By going with this stranger you have just made yourself an easy target for rape, murder, and abduction. My beautiful female if a stranger tells you your parents sent him (or her) to pick you up; go somewhere safe and call your parents. That way you can make sure they really sent this person to come and get you. If the stranger insists that you do not have to call your parents then you know to call the police because this person is trying to abduct you and harm you. Whatever you do; DO NOT go anywhere with that person.
If the stranger tries to grab you and make you go with him you scream as loud as you can, you bite that person as hard as you can, you scratch that person as hard as you can, you kick that person as hard as you can, you try to poke that person in the eye with your keys, you try to hit that person with anything you have or can get your hands on, you do whatever you need to do to get loose from that person. Once you get away you call the police right away so they can find this person and get him or her off the street and then you call your parents.

5th Safety Tip – Never accept a ride from a stranger.
If you were to accept a ride from a stranger there is a chance

that stranger may rape you, rob you, beat you, abduct you, or murder you. The stranger may even force you into prostitution. These things can take place all because you accepted a ride from a stranger.

GIVING MONEY TO STRANGERS

My precious female there will be times when you are approached by people you do not know who will ask you for some money. I want you to know you must be very careful when giving money to strangers. Giving money to strangers can be very dangerous. Going in your purse or pocket to give a stranger some money can lead to you being robbed by the very person that asked you for some money or by someone else who was watching you.

Another reason why you should not give money to strangers is you do not know who is in real need of your help. My beautiful female there are a lot of people pretending to be homeless, down on their luck, or handicap so people can give them their money. Since you do not know the intentions of the person who is asking for money I suggest you do not give any strangers any money; that way you can stay safe. Furthermore; no adult should be approaching a pre-teen or a teenage girl asking her for money.

SCAMS

My beautiful female there are a lot of different scams designed to take your money and steal your identity. These people are using the internet, the United States Postal Service, people, fake websites, and anything else they can think of to get you to give them your money and your personal information. List below are some of the different scams you should watch out for.

1st Scam – Check In The Mail

You will receive a check in the mail for several thousands of dollars attached with a letter saying congratulation this is a part of your winnings from a sweepstake. As you continue to read the letter it will tell you that all you have to do is send them money for the taxes via Money Gram, Western Union, or green dot prepaid visa card and they will release the rest of your money to you. My beautiful female do not send them any money. This is a scam.

What these con-artist are not telling you is that there is no sweepstakes and this is scam. The account the check is drawn on is a closed checking account. In some cases the check is drawn on a bank that does not exist. Listed below are more signs to let you know this is a scam.

1st Sign - You have to send money via Money Gram, prepaid visa card, or Western Union to get your money.

You must understand that once you wire the money to that person you will never get your money back. You will never receive the money from the sweepstake because there is no sweepstake. Plus, you will never be able to get in contact with that person once he or she receives your money.

My beautiful female any time you have to send someone some money so they can send you the money they have for you that is a scam.

2nd Sign – You did not enter any sweepstake.

My beautiful female how can you win a sweepstakes if you never entered one?

3rd Sign - A postal stamp was used on the envelope.

All legitimate businesses will have a postage machine which means they will not use postal stamps like the public use.

4th Sign – No return mailing address is listed on the envelope.

All legitimate businesses will list their business address on all of the mail they mail out.

2nd Scam – Phone Call
Soliciting Donations

My precious female another scam you should be aware of are people calling your phone asking for donations for firemen, police officers, Red Cross, United Way, Breast cancer association, National disaster victims fund, or any other nonprofit organization. None of these organizations will ever call your phone asking for donations.

The Fire Department and Police Department are not paid by donations. Therefore; they will not call you trying to solicit donations. Nonprofit organizations do receive some of their money from donations, but they never call people on the phone asking for donations. Nonprofit organizations have you mail it directly to their place of business. Plus, you are able to physically go to their place of business and make a donation.

The people who are calling you on your phone are trying to steal your banking information so they can steal money out of your checking account and savings account. Or they will try to get your visa card and master card number so they can make unapproved purchases with your credit card.

My precious female what you need to remember is that a legitimate business or nonprofit organization will not call you on your phone trying to solicit money from you. Especially, if you never made a donation to their foundation before.

3rd Scam – Phone Call From The IRS

My beautiful female there will be some people who will call your phone and tell you they are calling from the Internal Revenue Service (IRS). They will tell you that you owe back taxes and if you do not make a payment today they are going to send a sheriff to your home and even to your job to arrest you.

These con artists are calling you to try to get you to give them your your money. They will tell you can send the payment via electronic check, money gram, western union personal check, and even prepaid credit card.

First of all; my beautiful female, the IRS will never contact you by phone and request that you make a payment on your past do taxes. Nor will they send a sheriff to your house or to your job to arrest you if you do not make a payment over the phone.

Also, the Internal Revenue Service will send you documentation on their official letter head if there were any pass due taxes that you owed to the IRS.

If the IRS do not receive payment from someone who owes back taxes they will garnish that person's pay check or they will put a lien on that person's bank account, their property, or/and business. The IRS will never call you to make a payment over the phone or tell you to purchase a loadable prepaid debit card.

4th Scam – Email

My lovely female you will receive an email stating that you have a deceased relative who has millions and millions of dollars in a bank account in Africa and you are the sole survivor in the family. All they need for you to do is to send them your full name, complete mailing address, date of birth, social security number, and mother's maiden name and they can send you your money. By the way; everything they asked you to send them is everything you will need to apply for credit in the United States. Basically, this scam was created to steal your identity.

My beautiful female having your identity stolen can lead to you owing a lot of money to different companies. Also, because of that large amount of money that you owe you will not be able to get any credit from any financial institution. Or you may be charged with a crime you did not commit because the person gave the police your name, date of birth, and social security number.

If there really was a deceased person; who was a multi-millionaire, there would be a reading of a Will and Testament and not an email requesting this information from you. Listed below are some more signs to let you know that this is a scam.

1ˢᵗ Sign - You are named the sole survivor, but you have other blood relatives from both sides of your family who are alive.

2ⁿᵈ Sign – In order to get the money you have to give your full name, date of birth, complete mailing address, social security number, and mother's maiden name via email.

3ʳᵈ Sign – Thousands and thousands of people are getting the exact same email. Plus, none of those people are related to you by blood.

4ᵗʰ Sign - They never list the name of the deceased relative and his or her relationship to you.

5ᵗʰ Sign – You and your friend received the exact same email and you and your friend are not blood relatives.

BANKING

My precious female having a checking or savings account is a great accomplishment. It shows that you are mature and responsible enough to manage your own money. Not only do you need to be mature and responsible when having a bank account you need to be careful too. By being responsible and careful you are able to avoid some undesirable situations. Listed below are several tips you can follow to help you avoid undesirable situations while making transactions at your financial institution.

Safety Tips

1st Safety Tip - Never leave the teller's window
until you have put away your money.
By putting away your money before you leave the teller's window you will not draw attention to yourself because you are not exposing the cash you have just received. Plus, by putting away your money at the teller's window you are able to pay attention to your surroundings when you leave your financial institution.

2nd Safety Tip - Never leave the teller's window until you have put away all pieces of identification.
By putting away all pieces of identification before you leave the teller's window will minimize your chances of losing pieces of identification. Plus, by putting away all your identification at the teller's window you are able to pay attention to your surroundings when you leave your financial institution.

3rd Safety Tip – Always go to your financial

Lora McDuffie

institution with someone.
By having someone with you they can help you watch your surroundings. Also, being in a group of people lessen your chances
of getting rob.

CREDIT CARDS AND DEBIT CARDS

My precious female having a credit card or a debit card can make your life a lot simpler. Being able to access money and purchase things without having to go to a bank is a beautiful thing. Being in possession of this convenience it is up to you to make sure you protect your credit cards and debit cards.

Having you credit cards or debit cards in someone else's possession can lead to you having someone making unauthorized purchases with your credit cards or debit cards. Or they may take money out of your account or off your visa/master card.

Listed below are several things you can do to prevent someone from using your credit card or debit card to make purchases without your permission. Also, listed below are things you can do to keep people from taking money off of your card without your permission.

1ˢᵗ Thing - Never leave your credit card or debit card lying around the house.

By leaving your credit card or debit card out in the open it makes it easy for someone to steal your credit or debit card. Plus, they will be able to use your credit card or debit card because a lot of cashiers do not ask for identification when a purchase is being made.

2ⁿᵈ Thing – Do not leave your PIN (Personal Identification Number) number with your credit card or debit card.

By leaving your PIN number with your credit card or debit card the person who has your card now has your PIN number. Now that the person has your PIN number he or she is able to withdrawal money from your account at an ATM machine without your permission.

3rd Thing – Do not write your PIN number on the back of your credit card or debit card.

By writing your PIN number on the back of your credit card or debit card the person who has your card will be able to withdraw money from your account at an ATM machine or any retailer that allow you to get cash back with your purchase without your permission. Because you wrote your PIN number on the back of your card they can do transactions as a debit so they will not have to show identification while completing their transaction.

4th Thing – Select the credit cards or debit cards that allows you to have your picture printed on the front of the card.

By having your picture visible on the card retailer will be able to tell if the person presenting them the card is the actual card holder or a possible thief.

ATM CARDS

My lovely female having the ability to withdraw money at any time is a good thing. The convenience of going to an ATM versus going to the bank will save you time. Not only is it a good thing it can be a very dangerous thing. It is up to you to do everything you can to stay safe while using an ATM machine.

List below are several tips you can follow to stay safe while using an ATM machine.

Safety Tips

1st Safety Tip – Do not use an ATM machine at night.

By using an ATM machine at night you have just made yourself an easy target for a robbery because it is dark outside and a lot of people are not around. Plus, it is easier for someone to sneak up on you in the darkness.

2nd Safety Tip – Only use an enclosed ATM machines.

By using an ATM machine that is enclosed inside of a building it will give you a safer place to make your withdraw or deposit. Plus, those machines are equipped to not let another person to enter inside if it is occupied. Also, there are cameras inside and around the enclosed ATM.

3rd Safety Tip – Only use ATM machines that are in a well-lit area.

By using an ATM machine in a well-lit area you will be able to see what is going on around you and the people that are around will be able to see what is happening to you.

SHOPPING

My beautiful female there is nothing more exciting than going shopping. Buying things like clothes, shoes, jewelry, hand bags, perfume, or any other things you may buy can make you very happy, but there are people who want to steal your happiness away as well as the things you bought. Some of the thieves will steal your purse and even your car too. It is up to you to do everything you possible can to stay safe while shopping.
Listed below are several things you can do to stay safe while shopping.

Safety Tips

1st Safety Tip – Always go shopping with a buddy.
By shopping with a buddy you will have someone to help you watch your surroundings. Plus, thieves tend to target people who are by themselves and not paying attention to their surroundings. Also, if anything were to happen to you; and I hope it never does, the other person can go and get help.

2nd Safety Tip – Always keep a charged cell phone with you while shopping.
By having a charged cell phone you will be able to use your phone to take pictures of the person who victimized you, their license plate, and their car. That way you will be able to give the police information about your attacker. Also, you will be able to call 911 in case of an emergency. Plus, you will be able to call someone to come and pick you up in case you get stranded.

3rd Safety Tip – Do not pull your money out for everyone to see.

You should never pull your money out for everyone to see because some people will see your money and decide to rob you.

4th Safety Tip - Use a charge card or a debit card when shopping. Using a charge card or a debit card will not draw attention to you like using cash will.

5th Safety Tip – Do not leave your purse in
the shopping cart while shopping.
If you leave your purse in the shopping cart someone can walk up and steal it after you have walked away. Just so you know females will steal purses out of shopping carts too.

My lovely female when shopping during the major holidays like Easter, Thanksgiving, and Christmas you have to be extra careful. There are people who consciously wait for the Easter, Thanksgiving, and Christmas Season to rob people. These individuals pick these times of the year because people will be carrying a lot of cash with them to go shopping. It is up to you to be extra, extra careful during this time of the year.

Listed below are some things you can do to be safe while shopping during the major holiday seasons.

1st Thing – Do not carry very large hand bags.
Large hand bags are noticeable and it makes you an easy target for a purse snatcher.

2nd Thing – Do not put money in your purse.
If your money is not in your purse the individual who snatches your purse will not have your money.

3rd Thing – Wear your purse across your
body like a cross body bag.
It is a lot harder for someone to snatch your purse from you when you are wearing it across your body.

4th Thing – Valet your car if you are shopping for Christmas gifts.
By valeting your car you will not have to leave a secure area to get into your car. Plus, it is a lot safer to valet than versus walk-

ing through the park-N-lot during the holiday time.
If you decided to park in the park-N-lot during the Christmas Season; park your car in a lit area. That way you will be able to see everything around you.

5th Thing – Shop during the day time.
It is bright enough for you to see everything around.

6th Thing – Shop with a buddy.
By shopping with a buddy you will have someone to help you watch your environment

PAYING ATTENTION TO YOUR SURROUNDINGS

My beautiful female a lot of times females do not pay attention to their surroundings. Not paying attention to your surroundings makes you an easy target for predators. There predators are looking for unsuspecting females to rape, rob, carjack, abduct, or murder. Sometime these predators will do all five things to their victims.

You; my beautiful female, can avoid a lot of dangerous situations simply by being careful and paying attention to your surroundings. You should never let your guard down just because you are in a familiar neighborhood. Predators do not just stay in one area they travel around.

Listed below are some tips to keep you safe while you are out and about.

Safety Tips

1st Safety Tip – Avoid people who are dressed in clothes that are out of season.

For example: coats in the summer time, rain coats when it is not or have not been raining, gloves in the summer time, and knit ski mask in the summer time. Some people who wear clothes that are out of season are planning on robbing, raping, or murdering someone. In some cases they will use their clothes to conceal guns, knives, and sometimes bombs.

2nd Safety Tip – Always pay attention to the people around you. Some people will watch you and follow you in order to rob you, rape you, car jack you, abduct you, or murder you. Some predators will do all five things to their victims. That is why you need to pay attention to the people around you.

If you notice a particular person is always appearing everywhere you go you need to inform your parents so they can ask this individual why he or she is following you. Also, whenever possible; never go anywhere by yourself.

My beautiful female if you ever get the feeling that the person near you is unsafe to be around move away from them. My precious female never ignore what you are feeling; trust your instinct.

3rd Safety Tip – Never go home if you are being followed.

If you are driving your car and you notice someone is following you; do Not drive home. Drive to the nearest police station and call 911. Once you reach the police station blow your car horn so the police can come out the police station.

My beautiful female you should never drive home when you are being followed because the predator will know where you live and that opens the door for even more danger.

STRANGER FOLLOWING YOU IN HIS CAR

My beautiful female if ever you are walking down the street and someone pulls up and offers you a ride, drugs, or even money do not answer him (or her). By engaging in conversation you make yourself vulnerable to an attack. The more you respond to this stranger the more time you give him to carry out his plot to abduct you.

What you should do is turn around and go the opposite way; that way he cannot follow you. An even more effective way to avoid being abducted by a stranger following you in his car is to cross the street. By crossing the street the predator will not be able to drive along side of you because the flow of traffic is going in the opposite direction of where you are walking.

My precious female if ever you have to walk home, to work, or to the bus stop always walk opposite of the flow of traffic.

BEING BY YOURSELF

My lovely female there will be times when you will be by yourself. For those times when you are by yourself there are things you can do to keep yourself safe. Listed below are some tips you can follow to stay safe when you are by yourself.

Safety Tips

1st Safety Tip – Always take a charged cell phone with you
By having a charged cell phone you will be able to call 911 in case of an emergency. Plus, you will be able to contact someone to come and pick you up.

2nd Safety Tip – Never talk on your cell phone
while walking down the street by yourself.
When you are talking on your cell phone you are not fully paying attention to your surroundings. When you are not paying attention to your surroundings you become the perfect target for a robbery, an abduction, or even rape.

3rd Safety Tip – Always pay attention to your surroundings.
By paying attention to your surroundings you will be able to avoid some robberies as well as other undesirable situations.

4th Safety Tip – Do not take short cuts through alley.
If someone decides to rape you while you are walking through an alley no one will see you or hear you. Which means no one can help. If someone decides to rob you while you are walking through an alley no one will see you or hear you. Which means no one can help you.

5th Safety Tip – Do not talk on your cell phone

while walking down the street and night.
When you are talking on your cell phone you are not fully paying attention to your surroundings. When you are not paying attention to your surroundings you are the perfect target for a robbery, an abduction, or even rape.

USING PUBLIC TRANSPORTATION

My beautiful female not all of you will have vehicles you can drive when you need or want to go somewhere. Plus, there will be times when your parents and friends are not able to take you where you need or want to go; which means you may have to use public transportation. For those of you who have to use public transportation there are several things you can do to stay safe.

1st Thing – For those of you who pay your fare using cash I suggest you get the weekly, bi-weekly, or monthly buss pass. By using a bus pass you will not have to pull out money in front of people while waiting for public transportation. Since you are not pulling out money in front of people your chances of becoming a victim of robbery has just went down.

2nd Thing – When listening to your MP3 players, I Pods, or any other music devices DO NOT have the volume turned on high or on max volume. When you listen to these devices on a really high volume you are not able to hear what is going on around you. Now that you cannot hear what is going on around you; you have just become the perfect target for a rapist or robber. Plus, someone can sneak up on you and abduct you because you cannot hear him because of the loud music you are listening too.

3rd Thing – Do not talk on your phone while waiting for Public Transportation. When you are talking on the phone your focus will be on the

conversation and not what is going on around you. By not paying attention to your surroundings you can become the perfect
target for a robber, a rapist, or for someone to abduct.

THE DIFFERENCE BETWEEN BEING SCARED AND UNCOMFORTABLE

My precious female it is very important that you learn the difference between being scared and uncomfortable. Being scared is you not wanting to experience the outcome of your actions; even though you know what the outcome would be. By not wanting to experience the outcome of your actions it creates anxiety; that is what being scared is. In other words being scared is the anticipation of experiencing the outcome of your actions.

Being uncomfortable is something totally different. When you are uncomfortable about doing something that is not fear. That is a warning to let you know what you are about to do is not the best thing for you.

If you have any doubt or you are unsure about doing something you should not do it; that is a form of being uncomfortable. If you feel uneasy about doing something you should not do it; that is also a form of being uncomfortable. If you do not have peace about doing something you should not do it; that is a form of being uncomfortable too.

That uncomfortable feeling you get is placed inside you as a warning to keep you safe. If someone wants you to do something that makes you uncomfortable you should tell that person "No". If the person insists that you do it you can tell him or her very firmly "I Said No". Remember, my beautiful female; you do not have to do anything that makes you uncomfortable.

COOKING SAFETY

My beautiful female cooking can be very fun and exciting. Not only can you create something that will taste good you can create something that look very beautiful. I know cooking can be fun and exciting, but it can be very dangerous too. List below are some tips to keep you safe while cooking.

Tips To Stay Safe

1st Tip – Never put water on a grease fire.
If you were to use water to put out a grease fire it will cause the fire to spread and become uncontrollable. If ever you have a grease fire you can use baking soda or flour to put the fire out.

2nd Tip – Turn all pot handles and skillet handles inward on the stove when cooking.
By turning the handles inward on the stove you will not run into the handle and accidently spill hot food or hot liquid on yourself.

3rd Tips – Do not put a rug in front of the stove.
By having a rug in front of the stove you could slip on the rug and cause whatever food or liquid cooking on the stove to spill on you.

4th Tips – Never leave the house when you have food cooking on the stove.
By leaving the house you are unable to watch the food and the food can burn. Once the food has burned the next thing that will start burning is the pot or pan that you were cooking your food

in. If this was to happen the house or apartment you live in could catch on fire and burn down.

5th Tip – Do not put aluminum foil in the microwave.
If you put aluminum foil in the microwave you can cause the microwave to catch on fire.

6th Tip – Do not leave the house when you
have food cooking in the oven.
By leaving the house you are not able to watch the food and the food can burn. Once the food has burned the next thing to burn is the pan you have in the oven. If this was to happen the house or the apartment you live in can catch on fire.

7th Tip – Never leave a dish towel lying on the stove.
If a spark of fire gets on the dish towel the towel can catch on fire.

8th Tip – Do not stick silverware into the toaster
while it is plugged into the wall outlet.
By sticking silverware into the toaster you can cause yourself to get electrocuted.

9th Tip – Do not unplug any appliances with wet hands.
Using wet hands to unplug appliances can lead to you getting electrocuted.

10th Tip – Do not leave oven mitts on top of the stove.
If you leave oven mitts on top of the stove it can catch on fire.

11th Tip – Do not try to remove any pans, skillets, or
casserole dishes from the oven without and oven mitt
or a dish towel after the oven have been turned off.
Even though the food has not been cooking for a while the pan is still hot because the food in the pan is hot. Since the pan is still hot because of the food you will burn yourself. Plus, you may drop the pan of food on the floor. Now you have to deal with the burns you have on your hands and the mess you have on the

floor.

12th Tip – Always put your knives in the dish
rack with the blades facing downward.
By having the blade facing downward you will not accidentally
cut yourself when reaching in the dish rack.

13th Tip – Close all cabinet doors.
By keeping your cabinet doors closed you will not accidently
hit your head on the cabinet door.

14th Tip – Do not pour hot cooking oil into a plastic container.
If you pour hot cooking oil into a plastic container the container will melt and you will get burn by the hot oil spilling out.

15th Tip – Seek medical attention if you
cause a deep cut on your finger.
By not seeking treatment you can cause infection to set in the
wound. You may also loose sensation in that finger if not treated
immediately. Plus, the wound will not heal properly if you do
not get the stitches that are needed.

16th Tip – If you are cooking do not wear tops
that have long flowing sleeves.
Those flowing sleeves can accidentally catch on fire and cause
you to burn yourself.

17th Tip – When cooking never place a plate
on the stove lined with paper towel.
The paper towel can catch on fire.

18th Tip - Always make sure you turn the
oven off when you finish using it.
By double checking you can help avoid having gas seeping into
the air if you have a gas stove.

19th Tip – When frying food always make sure
you have your fire at medium heat.

By frying your food on medium heat you will cut down on your chances of getting burned by popping grease.

20th Tip – If you left silverware or a cooking utensil in the pot or pan you were cooking your food in do not try to remove the silverware or cooking utensil with your bare hand.
If you were to remove the silverware or cooking utensil with your bare hands you will burn your hands. That silverware of cook utensil has been heating up as the food was cooking.

21st Tip – Never put water in a glass dish you have removed from a heated oven.
By adding water to that glass dish you will cause that glass dish to shatter because of the drastic temperature change.

DRIVING

Getting your license is a very big accomplishment; not to mention very exciting. Now that you have your license you do not have to ask someone to take you to the movie. You do not have to ask someone to take you to work. You do not have to ask someone to take you to your friend's house. You do not have to ask someone to take you to your relative's house. All you have to do is get in the car and drive yourself whereever you want to go.

Not only do you have the freedom to go where you wanted to go you also have new responsibilities that comes with driving a car.

By not being responsible you can put yourself in several dangerous situations. My lovely female list below are some of the things you will need to be responsible for in order to be safe while driving.

1st Responsibility – Always make sure there is
at least a half a tank of gas in the car.
By not letting your gas tank go below a half a tank you will never run out of gas and become stranded.

2nd Responsibility – Always make sure you keep oil in your car.
By keeping oil in your car you can help prevent your engine from burning out. Plus, by keeping oil in your car your engine will not develop engine corrosion

3rd Responsibility – Always make sure you
have Anti-Freeze in your car.
By keeping Anti-Freeze in your car it will help prevent your car

from overheating. If your car over heats you will have engine problems. Having to replace your engine can cost you hundreds, and hundreds, and hundreds of dollars.

4th Responsibility – Always take your car
in for a tune up once a year.
By taking your car in for a tune up you can help your car to run better and last longer. Plus, a tune up can help you to locate minor mechanical problems before they become major mechanical problems.

5th Responsibility – Always leave a portable
car battery charger in your trunk.
By having a portable car battery charger you are able to use it whenever your battery dies. This will come in handy on those really cold winters and cold rainy days. Or on those days when you left your lights on and it drained your battery.

6th Responsibility – Always leave an ice scraper in your car.
By leaving an ice scraper in your car you will always have something to scrape the frost and ice off of your windshield at any given time it is needed.

7th Responsibility – Always leave a tire pressure gage in your car.
By having a tire pressure gage in your car you are able to check the pressure in your tire to make sure you did not over or under fill your tire with air. If you were to put too much air in your tires you can have a blowout while driving. If you did not put enough air in your tires it will cause you to burn more gas.

8th Responsibility – Always keep a flash light in your car.
When you have a flash light you can see what you are doing when you use your portable car battery charger. Plus, if ever you need to check something out under the hood and there is not enough light outside you can use your flash light to see what you are doing.

9th Responsibility– Always keep windshield
washer fluid in your car.
Having windshield washer fluid in your car can help you to keep your windshield clean and clear to look out of. When driving in the winter time other cars will splash the snow and salt mixture from the street, freeway, or highway on to your windshield. If you do not have windshield washer fluid and you use your windshield wipers it will smear the snow and salt mixture on your windshield and distort your view of the road. That distorted view of the road can possibly cause you to have an accident. By having windshield washer fluid in your car it will cut through the snow and salt mixture and leave your windshield clean and clear.

10th Responsibility – Always keep some
money with you when driving.
By having money with you; you will be able to put more gas in your car if needed.

My beautiful female while driving there are other steps you can take to keep yourself safe.

1st Step - Always wear your seat belt.
Wearing a seat belt can keep you from being thrown through the windshield if you are in a car accident. Also, wearing a seat belt can keep you from being tossed around in your car if you were in a rollover accident. In addition to the reasons previously listed it is the law and if the police pull you over for not wearing your seat belt you can and will get a ticket.

2nd Step – Do not text while driving.
Texting while driving can lead to you causing a car accident and killing someone. Or you can cause a car accident and kill yourself. If you were to text while driving you can crash your car into a tree or a building because you are not paying attention to the road. My beautiful female you must understand that those

few seconds that you have taken your eyes off the road can lead to a terrible car accident. Sometimes it can lead to a fatal car accident.

3rd Step – Do not drive drunk.
You should never drive drunk because your motor skills and reflexes will be slower than normal. Which means you will not be able to stop your car in enough time to not hit someone or something. Not only are your motor skills impaired so is your judgment. When your judgment is impaired you will not realize that you are speeding while driving. Now that you are speeding you may cause a car accident and possibly kill someone or even kill yourself. Also, you will not be able to stop your car in enough time to prevent hitting someone or something because your judgment is impaired.

In addition to all the reason previously listed it is against the law to drive drunk. If the police, state trooper, or sheriff pulls you over for driving drunk he or she can send you to jail and impound your car. The judge can suspend your license. Plus, your driver's record will list you as having a DUI - Driving under the Influence. Just so you know you can have your license suspended for years because you were driving drunk. Also, if you get a DUI on your driving record it will cause your insurance to be more expensive.

My beautiful precious female you need to know that if you are driving while drunk and you cause an accident and kill one of your passengers or all your passengers criminal charges can be filed against you. You can be charged with *MURDER* or *MAN SLAUGHTER*. It does not matter if it was an accident or even if your best friend was the one that died. You still will be charged with that person's death because you were driving while under the influence of alcohol.

4th Step – Do not go to the gas station at night by yourself.
By going to the gas station at night by yourself you have become

an easy target for a robbery or a carjacking. Simply because you are by yourself and it is dark outside.

5th Step – Always try to park your car in a well-lit area.
That way someone will always see you and your car. Also, if something was to happen to you; and I hope nothing ever does, you will be able to see your attacker because of the well-lit area you parked in. Plus, if someone was trying to sneak up on you; you will be able to see them because of the well-lit area you parked in.

6th Step – Always look in the window
before getting into your car.
My beautiful female you do not want to get into your car without looking in the window first because there could be someone lying on the back seat or on the floor waiting to rob you, carjack you, rape you, murder you, or do all four things listed above.

7th Step– Always pay attention to what
is going on around your car.
If you notice someone lingering around your car and you do not know that person he or she could be getting ready to steal something out your car or even steal your car. Or that person could be waiting on you so he or she could rob you.

My beautiful female if ever you notice someone lingering around your car you say in a very loud and firm voice "GET AWAY FROM MY CAR RIGHT NOW"!!!! Once that person moves away from your car then you get in your car, lock all your car doors, put on your seat belt, and drive away. If the person refuses to leave your car call the police and do not go to your car. You get as far away from your car and wait for the police.

8th Step – People lying on the ground by your car.
If you notice someone lying down on the ground beside your car do not go to your car. This person could be there waiting to rob you, rape you, carjack you, murder you, or do all four things to

you.

My beautiful female if ever you see someone lying beside your car do not try to get into your car. Go somewhere safe and ask someone to escort you to your car and wait for you to drive off to make sure you are safe.

9th Step – Do not drive fast through puddles of
water on the street, highway, or freeway.

By doing this you can cause your car to hydroplane on the sitting water. For those of you who do not know what hydroplane is it is your car taken flight because of the water you drove through.

Also you should not drive through any flooded area because the water could be deeper than you though cause your to stall out and have water damage.

10th Step – Do not dial your phone while driving.

When you look at your phone to dial someone; you take your eyes off the road. By taking your eyes off the road just for a few seconds you can cause an accident and KILL someone or even KILL yourself.

11th Step – Never drive while high on drugs;
that includes prescription drugs.

You should never drive while high on drugs because your motor skills and reflexes are slower than normal when you are high. Which means you will not be able to stop your car in enough time in order to not hit someone or something. Also, your judgment will be impaired. Now that your judgment is impaired you will not realize that you are speeding or drifting into another lane. If you are speeding or drifting into another lane you may cause a car accident.

Another reason why you should never drive while high on drugs is because the police can pull you over for driving while under the influence. The officer can impound your car and send you to jail. The judge can suspend your license and your driving record will list you as having a DUI - Driving under the Influence. Just so you know you can have your license suspended for years because you were driving while under the influence of drugs. Also, if you get a DUI on your driving record it will cause your insurance to be even more expensive.

My precious female you need to know if you are driving while high on drugs and you cause and accident and kill one of your passengers or all of your passengers criminal charges can be filed against you. The charges that will be filed against you will be *Murder* or *Man Slaughter*. It does not matter if it was an accident or if it was your best friend or family member that died; you still will be charged with that person's death because you were driving while high on drugs.

12th Step – Do not put on makeup while driving.
When you are putting on makeup you will use your mirror to see what you are doing; which mean you are not focusing on the road. Since you are not paying attention to the road you can cause an accident and kill someone.

13th Step – Always lock your car doors once inside your car.
By locking your car doors no one can walk up to your car, open the door, and take your purse and other item out the car. No one will be able to open your car door and snatch you out the car so they carjack you. By having your car doors lock a guy cannot open the door and enter into your car and force you to drive him somewhere at gun point so he can rape you.

14th Step – Do not leave valuables visible inside your car.
Having your valuables visible in your car can encourage a thief to break into your car to steal your things. Now you will have to replace the items that were stolen as well as replace the broken window too.

My beautiful female you need to know that your car can be broken into in the suburbs as well as in the inner city. You must understand that a thief does not have restrictions on where he or she can steal from.

15th Step – Do not drive while you are sleepy.
If you drive while you are sleepy; you can fall asleep at the wheel and crash your car into a tree. Or you can fall asleep at the wheel and hit someone and injure that person or even kill that person.

16th Step – Do not take selfies (pictures of you) while driving.
When taking selfies while driving your attention is not fully focused on the road and that can be very dangerous. By not focusing on the road you can cause a car accident and possibly injure or kill someone. You may even kill yourself in that car accident all because you were taking selfies.

RIDING IN A CAR WITH FRIENDS

My beautiful female if you are riding in a car with your friend and he or she is speeding it is up to you to tell your friend to slow down. Do not sit there and be quite if your friend is driving recklessly while you are riding in the car. Their reckless driving can cause and accident that can lead to you having your legs or arms amputated, you can become paralyzed, or you can die.

If your friend always drives recklessly everytime you ride with him; or her, it is up to you to decide if riding in the car with your friend worth you becoming an amputee, paralyzed, or dead.

GOING TO THE NIGHT CLUB

My lovely female as you get older you will start going to the night clubs with your friends. Going to the night club can be so much fun. You get to dress up, hang out with your friends, meet new people, and have a lot of fun. Even though going to the night club can be a lot of fun it can also be very dangerous. Listed below are some tips you can follow to stay safe while at the club.

Safety Tips

1st Tip – Always go to the night club with friends.
By going with your friends you will have someone to watch out for you while you are at the night Plus, you will not have to walk to your car by yourself in the dark. Also, you will have someone there to help protect you if something was to happen.

2nd Tip – Always carry a charged cell phone with you.
By having a charged cell phone you will be able to call 911 if there is an emergency. Also, you will be able to call someone to come and pick you up if it became unsafe for you to let your friend drive you home. Plus, you can call your friend to find out where she is in case you both get separated.

3rd Tip – Only accept drinks from a waitress or waiter.
The guy could have put GHB, Rohypnol, Ketamine, a tranquilizer, or any other debilitating drug in your drink. If you were

to drink that drink it will cause you to be incoherent or non-responsive to what is going on around you or to you. If this was to happen to you it will make it easier for the guy to rape you, rob you, murder you, abduct you, or do all four things to you.

4th Tip – Never accept candy from people at
the night club you do not know.
The candy you are eating may not be candy, but drugs. Taking those drugs can put you in several undesirable situations because your judgment will be impaired because of the drugs you have taken. The drugs you have taken; because you thought it was candy, may cause you to have a heart attack, brain damage, or even seizures. In some cases the drug you have taken may kill you.

5th Tip – Never leave the night club with a guy you
just met and go to his house or apartment.
Going back to the guy's house after you just met him can lead to you being raped, robbed, or even murdered.

6th Tip – Never drink a drink you have left unattended.
Your drink may have been spiked with a Date Rape Drug, a tranquilizer, or any other debilitating drug. Those drugs can make you incoherent and nonresponsive to what is going on around you or to you. Once you are in this state of mind the person who spiked your drink can rape you, rob you, murder you, abduct you, or your attacker can do all four things to you.

SPRING BREAK

My lovely female going away for Spring Break can be very exciting. You get to hang out with your friends, make new friends, go to a different state, a different country, or even a different continent, and there are NO PARENTS. Now that you have absolute freedom to do what you want, when you want. You also have the full responsibility of keeping yourself safe while away for Spring Break. My beautiful female there are several things you can do to stay safe while away for Spring Break.

Safety Tips

1st Safety Tip – Never go anywhere by yourself.
By having someone with you at all times you will always have someone looking out for you.

2nd Safety Tip – Never accept rides from guys you do not know.
Accepting a ride from a stranger in another state, country, or continent can be very dangerous. This guy can rape you, rob you, murder you, abduct you, or do all four things to you.

You must know that there are people who prey on tourist. They believe that if they were to commit a criminal act against a tourist there is a greater chance that the victim will not press charges against them. Simply because the victim do not live there and the victim will never have to see their attacker again.

Just so you know people will know you are a tourist because your dialect would be different, the way you dress would be different, and the excitement of being in a new place. All these things are indicators that you are not from the area. My beautiful female if someone commit a criminal act against you please file a police report against your attacker. What this person did is wrong and he or she should be held accountable for their actions.

3rd Safety Tip – Do not accept drinks from
anyone other than a waitress or waiter.
A drink given to you by someone other than a waitress or waiter may be spiked with GHB, Rohypnol, Ketamine, a tranquilizer, or any other debilitating drug. The person who spikes a female's drinks usually plans on raping, robbing, abducting, or murdering her. In some case the person may do all four things to their victim. So if you did not have a waitress or waiter bring you your drink I suggest you DO NOT drink that drink. Better safe than sorry.

4th Safety Tip – Do not get drunk.
By getting drunk you make yourself an easy target for a rapist, a robber, an abductor, or even a murderer. Just so you know it takes less alcohol to get a female drunk than it does for a male.

5th Safety Tip – Never leave your friend to go
somewhere with a guy you just met.
By leaving with a guy you just met you will be putting yourself at risk of being raped, beaten, robbed, abducted, or murdered. In some cases the guy will do all five things to you.
If you want to spend time with a guy you just met; hang out with him with your friends. That way your friends can watch out for you as well as watch him too.

6th Safety Tip – Always keep a charged cell phone with you.
If you were to get separated from your friends you will be able to call your friends to find out where they are so you can meet back up with them. Also, you will be able to call 911 if ever there is an emergency.

7th Safety Tip – Agree to board the bus,
airplane, or train together.
By making this agreement you and your friends will be able to
make sure everyone get home safely. If your friends do not show
up when it is time to board the bus, airplane, or train, you will
know that something is wrong and you will know to contact
the police.

8th Safety Tip – Get to know the people
you meet and hang out with.
By gathering information about the guys and females you and
your friends are hanging out with; you will have some information to give to the police if anything was to happen to you or any
of your friends.

9th Safety Tip – Call your friends approximately
two hours before it is time to return home.
By calling your friends you are able to make sure they are up
and getting ready to leave. It will keep them from missing their
flight, the bus, or the train. Also, if you call your friends and you
get no answer you can call the front desk so they can check to
see if they are ok.

10th Safety Tip – Always trust your instinct.
If you meet a guy (or female) and you get the feeling that he (or
she) is unsafe to hang out with TRUST YOUR INSTINCT. That uncomfortable feeling you get is placed inside you to protect you
from harm and danger.

11th Safety Tip – Never accept candy from
a guy you met at Spring Break.
The candy you are accepting could be drugs.

12th Safety Tip – Call your parents or guardian
when you get to your destination.
That way your parents will know that you made it safely.

13th Safety Tip - Make sure you program in your
phone the name, the address, and the phone number
of the hotel where you will be staying.
By having the hotel information stored in your phone you will
always have it in case you cannot remember it.

14th Safety Tip – Give your parents or someone
you trust the name, address, and phone number
of the hotel where you will be staying.
By giving your parents or someone you trust the information to
the hotel they will be able to notify you in case there is an emergency at home. Or if they need to come to you they will know
where to go.

TATTOOS

Tattoos are beautiful and permanent works of art for the body. Some people get tattoos to help them visually express their individuality. Some people get tattoos to remember a special occasion in their life. Some people get tattoos to commemorate the life or death of a love one. Tattoos are a permanent way to remind oneself of something or someone.

For those of you who do not know what takes place when you get a tattoo let me explain it to you. When getting a tattoo the tattooist is making hundreds of punctures into your skin with a needle. With each puncture of the needle dye is placed under the top layer of your skin (the Dermis). The dye is what creates the tattoo that you want.

My beautiful female because of the puncture wounds you get in order to get your tattoo your body has become susceptible to blood borne diseases. List below are some of the blood borne disease you may contract.

- Syphilis
- Hepatitis
- Tetanus
- Tuberculosis
- Human Immunodeficiency Virus (HIV)
- Herpes Simplex Virus

If the needle the tattooist used to give you your tattoo was used on someone who has contaminated blood; that blood will be transferred to your blood. Once that contaminated blood comes in contact with your blood; your blood will become contaminated.

If your blood was to become contaminated with the Syphilis

Virus you can experience blindness, mental illness, heart diseases, and even death.

If your blood was to become contaminated with the Human Immunodeficiency Virus (HIV) it will gradually destroy your immune system. Once your immune system is completely destroyed you will develop AIDS (Acquired Immune Deficiency Syndrome). Now that you have the AIDS Virus your body will deteriorate at an alarming rate and you will eventually die.

As you can see; getting a tattoo can lead to you contracting a blood borne disease such as Syphilis, Hepatitis, Tetanus, Tuberculosis, Herpes Simplex Virus, or even Human Immunodeficiency Virus (HIV) if proper precautions are not taken.

My precious female if you do decide to get a tattoo be sure to go to a licensed professional. Also, make sure that a brand new needle is used to give you your tattoo. Do not under any circumstance allow a tattooist to use a used need on you; it does not matter if it is a family member or a close friend. If the tattooist does not want to use a new needle do not allow that person to give you your tattoo. Your life and health is more important than that tattoo you are about to put on your body.

DOWN POWER LINES

My precious one there will be times when you will come across a down power line. Sometimes those down power lines will be shooting out sparks letting you know that it is a live wire (still full of electrical current). In some cases you will not see sparks coming from a down power line, but that power line will still be considered as a live wire because there is still an electrical current in the wire. I want you to know if you were to touch a live wire or even step on a live wire you will get electrocuted. If your body was to get shocked by hundreds and hundreds of currents of electricity you may suffer from brain damage, permanent body damage, or even death. You must understand that touching or stepping on a down power line may lead to your death.

VAGINA

My beautiful female your vagina is a very sensitive part of your body and it is up to you to do whatever you can to protect it from being irritated or getting an infection.

Knowing What Your Vagina Looks Like

My precious female it is very important that you know what your vagina looks like. I suggest you take a mirror and take a good look at your vagina. Pay attention to the color, the shape, and the thickness of the small and large labium (lips). By knowing what your vagina looks like when it is healthy you will notice if there is any changes in your vagina due to Bacterial Vaginosis or any other vaginal infections you may have.

My beautiful female; make sure that your hands and finger nails are clean when you take a mirror and look at your vagina. Plus, if you ever notice anything that does not look right please visit your gynecologist. If you do not have one I suggest you select one.

TOXIC SHOCK SYNDROME

My precious one; if you are using tampons be sure to change your tampons often. That way you can avoid developing *Toxic Shock Syndrome* (TSS). For those of you who do not know what Toxic Shock Syndrome is; it is a toxic infection that can be life threatening. The Bacteria that causes Toxic Shock Syndrome is *Staphylococcus Bacteria.* If ever you become infected with the *Staphylococcus Bacteria* you will need to seek medical attention immediately. Some of the symptoms you can experience from Toxic Shock Syndrome are:
- Sudden fever over 102 degrees
- Vomiting
- Diarrhea
- Muscle aches
- Stomach cramps
- Low blood pressure
- Rapid heartbeat
- Fainting
- Feeling lightheaded
- Confusion
- Body rash resembling a sun burn

If Toxic Shock Syndrome (TSS) goes untreated it can lead to seizures and multiple organ failure.

For those of you who still do not understand what Toxic Shock Syndrome is let me explain it to you this way. The blood that is absorbed in the tampon that you are wearing can cause a bacterial infection inside your vagina if the tampon has been worn for

Lora McDuffie

a long period of time. The bacteria that causes Toxic Shock Syndrome is called *Staphylococcus Bacteria* and it can be life threatening. To avoid developing Toxic Shock Syndrome change your tampons frequently or use sanitary napkins.

VAGINAL IRRITATION

My beautiful female you should be aware of the things that can cause you to experience vaginal irritation. When you develop vaginal irritation it can be very uncomfortable. Some of the symptoms you can experience are:
- Vaginal dryness
- Itching
- Burning
- Not being able to wear panties because anything touching your vagina irritates it even more
- Burning while urinating
- Stinging while urinating
- Swollen vaginal lips
- Thick white discharge resembling cottage cheese
- Discharge having a fishy odor

Some of the things that can cause you to experience vaginal irritation are listed below.

Dye In Panties

One thing that you should be aware of that can cause vaginal irritation is the dye that is used for dying panties. Some panties that are dyed bleed and when the dye comes in contact with the vagina it can cause your vagina to become irritated. If your vagina becomes irritated from the dye that is used to dye panties that can be one of the most uncomfortable feeling you will experience. Listed below are some tips to help you avoid vaginal irritation from the dye used to dye panties.

Tips To Avoid Vaginal Irritation From Dye In Panties

1st Tip – Buy panties that have white cotton crotches.

2nd Tip - If you buy red or black panties be sure to wash them before you wear them; these color panties are usually the ones that bleeds.

3rd Tip – Wash all colored panties before wearing them.

4th Tip – Wear panty liners with all panties that do not have a white cotton crotch.

If you were to experience vaginal irritation from the dye used to dye panties you can sit and soak in a tub of cool water and it should bring you some relief.

Wearing Panties That Are Too Small

Another thing that can cause your vagina to become irritated is wearing panties that are too small. When you wear your panties too small the constant friction of your panties rubbing against your vagina and going inside your vagina can cause your vagina to become very dry. Because your vagina is dry along with the constant rubbing this is where the irritation comes from. So my beautiful female make sure you buy your panties the right size so you will not have to experience any discomfort.

How To Tell If Your Panties Are Too Small

1st Indication – If the elastic around your thigh is extremely tight.

2nd Indication – If your panties constantly go inside your vagina whenever you move or walk.

3rd Indication – If your panties continually separate at the seams.

4th Indication – When the elastic on the waist band and thigh is stretched to its full capacity.

5th Indication – If the elastic waist band separate from the rest of the panty.

6th Indication – If the elastic around the leg opening separates from the rest of the panty.

My beautiful female if you are experiencing any of the things listed above you should purchase your panties in a larger size.

Perfume In Products

My beautiful female another thing that can cause vaginal irritation is the perfume that is used in some products such as: soaps, shower gels, body wash, douches, bath oils, and bubble bath. Because every beautiful female's vagina holds its own level of sensitivity, you my beautiful female; will have to determine what can be used and what cannot be used to clean your vagina.

Tips To Avoid Vaginal Irritation From Perfume In Products

1st Tip – Buy products that are made for sensitive skin.

2nd Tip – Avoid products that states fragrance added.

3rd Tip – Avoid products that have a very strong perfume scent.

4th Tip – Use products that have all natural ingredients.

If you were to experience vaginal irritation from the perfume in soaps, shower gels, body washes, douches, or bubble baths you can sit and soak in a tub of cool water and it should bring you some relief.

Making Bubble Baths Or Taking Showers Using Anti-Bacterial Dish Washing Liquid

For those beautiful females who use anti-bacteria dish washing liquid to create a bubble bath or to take a shower with you should know that anti-bacteria products kill bacteria. Plus, anti-bacterial products strip the moisture from the body part it comes in contact with. By having the moisture removed from the vagina as well as altering the bacteria levels that are found inside the vagina you will cause yourself to experience vaginal irritation.

One way you can tell if a particular product is irritating your vagina is shortly after using that product you may begin to experience:

- Intense itching
- Burning
- Stinging
- Burning when urinating
- Stinging when urinating
- Some swelling of the vagina
- Vaginal dryness

Tip For Avoiding Vaginal Irritation From Using Anti-Bacterial Dish Washing Liquid For Bubble Bath Or Taking Showers

1st Tip – Use bubble bath to make a bubble baths.

2nd Tip – Use shower gel for taking showers

If you ever experience vaginal irritation from using Anti-Bacterial dish washing liquid you can sit and soak in a tub of cool water and it should bring you some relief.

Bacterial Vaginosis And Yeast Infections

My lovely female you should be aware of the things that can cause you to experience Bacterial Vaginosis or a yeast infection. Some of the symptoms you can experience from Bacterial Vaginosis and a yeast infection are:

- A thick white discharge that look like cottage cheese
- Itching (sometimes very intense itching)
- Stinging when urinating
- A foul odor
- Burning when urinating

- Unable to wear panties because anything touching your vagina causes more irritation.
- The lips of the vagina will be swollen
- Vaginal dryness
- Discharge with a foul odor or fishy odor

Listed below are some things that can cause you to experience Bacterial Vaginosis or a yeast infection.

Wearing Panties Made Out Of Synthetic Fabrics

Wearing panties made out of synthetic fabric may cause you to experience Bacterial Vaginosis or a yeast infection. Panties made out of synthetic fabrics will hold in heat and moisture from your vagina. When the heat and moisture is unable to escape because of the non-breathable fabrics it will cause the *Anaerobic Bacteria* in the vagina to grow. The multiplying of the Anaerobic Bacteria will cause you to have Bacterial Vaginosis or a yeast infection.

Tip To Avoid Bacterial Vaginosis And Yeast Infection From Panties Made Out Of Synthetic Fabrics

1st Tip – Wear panties made out of cotton or natural fabrics that breathe.

2nd Tip – If you want to still wear panties made out of synthetic fabrics make sure the panties have a white cotton crotch.

Wearing Really Tight Pants

My beautiful female when you wear really tight pants the heat and moisture from your vagina is unable to escape. When the heat and moisture is unable to escape it will causes the Anaerobic Bacteria in the vagina to grow and multiply. The multiplying of the Anaerobic Bacteria will cause you to develop Bacterial Vaginosis or a yeast infection.

Tips To Avoid Bacterial Vaginosis And Yeast

Lora McDuffie

Infections From Wearing Tight Pants

1st Tip – Wear pants that are not tight.

WAXING

My beautiful female there will be some of you who will wax your body so you can have smooth hairless skin. If you choose to wax parts of your body there are several things you can do to protect your body from harm and damage due to waxing.

1ˢᵗ Thing – Do not wax irritated, sun burned, or broken skin.
By waxing irritated, sun burned, or broken skin you can cause the irritated area to become even more irritated.

2ⁿᵈ Thing – Make sure the wax is not over heated.
If the wax is too hot your skin can become discolored and burned. You will also have reddish brown spots on your skin because you have *Post Inflammatory Pigmentation* due to the over-heated wax you applied on your skin. Just so you know it can take anywhere from a week to a year for your skin to heal and become its natural color.

3ʳᵈ Thing – If your skin becomes irritated and red after waxing apply ice on the irritated area.
The ice will help reduce the irritation.

4ᵗʰ Thing – If you begin to have an allergic reaction to the products used to wax your body seek medical attention.

5ᵗʰ Thing – If you are using or taking any products with vitamin A such as; Retin-A, Renova, Diffferin, Accutane, or Isoretinoin you should avoid getting your body waxed. Products with vitamin A in it can cause tearing of the skin.

My beautiful female there are other side affects you can experience from getting your body waxed. For instance:
- Ingrown hair (hair curling up under your skin producing hair

bumps)
- Loss of skin radiance with long term waxing
- Loss of elasticity of skin with long term waxing
- Developing wrinkles with long term waxing
- Develop skin rashes, reddish bumps, and light bleeding

MOLESTATION

My precious one I want you to know that no one has the right to touch your body in a sexual way or in any other way that makes you uncomfortable; not your father, not your mother, not your grandfather, not your grandmother, not your brother, not your sister, not your half-sister, not your half-brother, not your uncle, not your aunt, not your cousin, not your friends, not your friend's parents, not a friend of the family, not your neighbors, not a pastor, not a priest, not the deacon of the church, not a bishop, not an arch diocese, not a reverend, not the elders of the church, not a teacher, not coach, not counselor, not even a stranger.

I need you to understand that anyone can be a molester; a grown man, a grown woman, someone younger than you (a boy or a girl), someone who is bigger than you, someone smaller than you, someone who is just a few years older than you, or someone your age.

If a guy is touching your breast, vagina, buttock, or any other part of your body in a sexual way or a way that makes you uncomfortable he is wrong for doing that and you should tell an adult. If a guy is asking you to touch him in a sexual way or in a way that makes you uncomfortable he is wrong for doing that and you should tell an adult. If a guy is touching on himself and he is asking you to watch him while he masturbates he is wrong for doing that and you should tell an adult. If a guy is forcing you to perform oral sex on him he is wrong for doing that and you should tell an adult. If a guy is forcing you to allow him to perform oral sex on you he is wrong for doing that and you should tell an adult. If a guy is forcing you to have sex with him he is wrong for doing that and you should tell an adult. That way you will have someone to go to the police station with you to file a police report against your abuser.

My beautiful female; if any of these things are happening to you or have happened to you please tell an adult. If the adult you told do not believe you; you need to tell another adult and you keep telling until someone believes you. If there are no adult you can tell you can tell the police; the ministers at your church, or a teacher, or even the principal at your school.

You must understand that men are not the only ones that can molest you, women can molest you too. Whether it is a male or a female who is molesting you that person is wrong for violating you sexually.

My beautiful female some molesters will make the things that they are doing to you feel pleasurable. The pleasure that you are feeling is not because you like what he or she is doing to you, but because your body is sensitive to touch and stimulation. That is why your molester is doing what he or she is doing to you. Your molester is aware of the fact that your body is sensitive to touch and stimulation. Your predator is hoping you felt some pleasure from what he was doing to you that way you will feel guilty and not tell on him or her. Some predators will use the guilt and fear that their victim is feeling as a tool to keep them from telling. I am asking you to be brave and tell, tell, and tell again. You need to tell someone so they can get this person away from you and keep this person from molesting you.

It is not your fault why this person chose to molest you. It is not your fault that this molester chose to violate you sexually. There is nothing you could have done differently to prevent this from happening to you. This person was going to molest you no matter what you did or did not do. You need to know that you did absolutely nothing wrong. There is nothing wrong with you and you have nothing to be ashamed of. The person who is molesting you or who had molested you that person should feel ashamed because he violated you sexually for his own sexual gratification.

My precious female if this was to ever happen to you or if it had happened in the past please tell someone. I know it will be difficult, but you are a strong and brave female and you can do it. Once you tell someone you can begin to heal from this horrible thing that has happened to you.

My beautiful female some molesters usually test and prep their victims before they take it to sexual intercourse. List below are some of the things molesters do.

One thing some molesters will do is convince their victims that they are trust worthy. These molesters will do this by being very kind and friendly to their targeted victim. They will spend time talking and listening to the person they plan on molesting. They will give things and gifts to their victim in order to make them feel special. The molesters will even give their victim a pet name or nick name because he wants them to believe they are very special to him.

My lovely female if ever you begin to feel that something is not right about a person TRUST YOUR INSTINCT. Your instincts are there to protect you from harm and danger and that includes molesters too. You do not have to spend time with someone you do not trust even if it is a family member or a friend of the family. If you do not trust someone who always try to spend time with you tell your parents that you do not feel safe around this person and tell them why. Then ask them to please keep that person away from you.

Another thing that some molesters will do is try to spend a lot of time alone with their targeted victim. Spending time alone with his victims is very important because the molester need the victim to be comfortable with being around him without someone else around. It will be at this time when the molester will try different things to see if their targeted victim will allow him to do those things to her.

One of the things molesters will do is kiss their victim on their forehead, the top of their head, and on their cheek to get her use to having him kissing on her. What will eventually happen is one day the molester will kiss his targeted victim on the lips.

After kissing his victim he will wait to see what her response will be. What this molester is waiting to see is if their targeted victim will respond as if she is offended and about to tell. Or will his targeted victim freeze up and not say anything because what the predator did made her very uncomfortable. The molester is hoping that his targeted victim would freeze up and not say or do anything. If this happens the predator will be able to kiss his victim on the lips again.

My beautiful female if ever you begin to feel that something is not right about a person TRUST YOUR INSTINCT. Your instincts are there to protect you from harm and danger and that includes molesters too.

Another thing that some molesters will do is brush their hand or arm across their targeted victims breast, buttock, or vagina. What these molesters are doing is trying to see if they can get away with touching their targeted victim's breast, buttock, or vagina. Once the molester realizes that their target victim is not going to say anything he will begin to touch them on a regular basis.

These are a few things that some molesters will do in order to test and prep their victims before they take it to sexual intercourse.

My beautiful female letting a molester touch and feel on you with the hope that he will never ever ask again is not a good idea; even if he tells you he will never ask again. You must know a molester will lie to you to get what he wants. I want you to know you do not have to let a molester touch and feel on you in order to get him to leave you alone. You need to realize that once you let a molester touch and feel on you he will do it whenever an opportunity presents itself. Once the predator is able to touch your body purposely the next thing he will try to do is have sex with you.

My precious female you do not have to spend time with someone who is molesting you. Or someone who makes you uncomfortable because of the way he touches you and looks at you.

If someone is touching you in a sexual way or in a way that

makes you uncomfortable you tell that person in a very firm and loud voice DO NOT TOUCH ME EVER AGAIN!!! I do not care if it is a grown man, a grown woman, a family member, a family friend, a stranger, or even somebody younger than you; you tell them very firmly and loudly DO NOT TOUCH ME EVER AGAIN!!! I know it can be very scary to do this, but I want you to know that you are a strong and brave beautiful female and you can do this. Once you do this please tell your parents or guardian what happened so they can keep this molester away from you.

Remember, my beautiful female; this is your body and no one and I mean no one has the right to touch your body without your permission. Plus, you do not have to do anything that makes you uncomfortable nor do you have to be around people who make you uncomfortable.

My beautiful female you must understand and know it is never your fault if someone molest you. You did not do anything to cause him to molest you. Plus, it is not your fault why this predator chose to violate you sexually.

NOW YOU KNOW

CLOSING

My beautiful female I hope the information that I have shared with you in this book help to keep you safe while you explore life.

CONTACT INFORMATION

If you would like to leave a comment or a brief message for the author you can email Lora McDuffie at: straight_talk4girls@yahoo.com

REFERENCE

Cellulitis, Retrieved from http://www.medicinenet.com/cellulitis/article.htm

Heroin, Retrieved from http://www.drugs.com/heroin.html

Heroin, Retrieved from http://www.drugfree.org/Portal/Drug_guide/Heroin

Heroin, Retrieved from http://www.treatment4addiction.com/drugs/narcotics/heroin/

Heroin, Retrieved from http://en.wikipedia.org/wiki/Heroin

Ketamine Effects, Retrieved from http://www.thegooddrugsguide.com/ketamine/effects.htm

Governments moves to control Ketamine, Retrieved from http://www.ketamine.com/legal.html

KETAMINE THE ULTIMATE PSYCHEDELIC JOURNEY, Retrieved from http://www.ketamine.com/dmturner/index.html

What is Ketamine, Retrieved from http://www.thegooddrugsguide.com/ketamine/index.htm

What Every Female Should Know By Age 21, Retrieved from http://voices.yahoo.com/what-every-female-know-age-21-12171146.html

Ketamine, Retrieved from http://www.theantidrug.com/drug-information/commonly-abused-drugs/ketamine.aspx

McDuffie, L. (2009) *Dating: What Every Pre-teen And Teenage Girl Should Know.*
Baltimore MD: Publish America

Ketamine (Ketalar), Retrieved from http://micro.magnet.fsu.edu/pharmaceuticals/pages/ketamine.html

ECSTASY EFFECTS, Retrieved from http://www.ecstasyeffects.net/Ecstasy_Safe_Effects.htm

MDMA, Retrieved from http://www.erowid.org/chemicals/mdma_basics.shtml

MDMA, Retrieved from http://en.wikipedia.org/wiki/MDMA

Ketamine, Retrieved from http://en.wikipedia.org/wiki/Ketamine
UTOPIAN PHARMACOLOGY Mental Health in the Third Millennium MDMA and Beyond, Retrieved from http://www.mdma.net/
http://health.rutgers.edu/brochures/ecstacy.htm

Ecstasy, Retrieved from http://www.cesar.umd.edu/cesar/drugs/ecstasy.asp

Effects of MDMA on the human body, Retrieved from http://en.wikipedia.org/wiki/
Effects_of_MDMA_on_the_human_body

McDuffie, L. (2010) *Sex & STD's: What Every Pre-teen And Teenage Girl Should Know.*
Baltimore MD: Publish America

Ketamine, Retrieved from http://www.projecghb/ketamine.htm

Ketamine, Retrieved from http://www.abovetheinfluence.com/facts/drugs-ketamine.aspx?id=search_properKetamine

Dissociative Anaesthetics KETAMINE (Ketalar, Vetalar, Ketacet, Ketajet), Retrieved from http://www.ketamine.com/dissociative-anaesthetic.html

Dissociative Anaesthetics KETAMINE (Ketalar, Vetalar, Ketacet, Ketajet), Retrieved from http://www.justice.gove/ndic/pubs4/4769/index.htm

Ketamine, Retrieved from http://wwwdrugfree.org/Portal?Drug_guide?ketamine

Ketamine, Retrieved from http://www.druginfo.adf.org.au/druginfo/drugs/drugfact/ketamine.html

Ketamine Addiction, Retrieved from http://www.drugrehab.net/2009/09/12/ketamine-abuse/

HEROIN ADDICTION, Retrieved from http://www.heroin-addiction.info/side-effects.htm

Marijuana Side Effects, Retrieved from http://www.personalhealthzone.com/marijuanasideeffects.html

How bad is marijuana for you, Retrieved from http://wiki.answer.com/Q/How_bad_is_marijuana_for_you

Marijuana addiction, Retrieved from http://www.marijuana-addiction.info/side-effects.htm

Marijuana Addiction, Retrieved from http://www.treatment4addiction.com/addiction/marijuana

Weed out marijuana use, Retrieved from http://drug-abuse.suite101.com/article.cfm/weed_out_marijuana_use http://www.freepublic.com/focus/f-news/1933486/post

Marijuana, Retrieved from http://www.drugfree.org/Portal?Drug_guide/Marijuana

Marijuana, Retrieved from http://www.acde.org/common/Marijuana.htm http://Kidshealth.org/teen/drug_alcolol_tobacco/smoiking.html

Smoking Diseases, Retrieved from http://www.quit-smoking-stop.com/smoking-diseases.html

Smoking, Retrieved from http://www.smoking-ceassation.org/content/healthissues.asp

Just how does smoking harm my health?, Retrieved from http://www.silkquit.org/stop-smoking/as3faq/how-does-smoking-harm-my-health.aspx

Smoking Statistics – Tobacco Use and How it Affects Us, Retrieved from http://quitsmoking.about.com/od/tobaccostatistics/a/CigarettesSmoke.htm

Cigarette Smoking, Retrieved from http://www.youngwomenshealth.org/smokeinfo.html

Smoking, Retrieved from http://kidshealth.org/teen/drug_alcohol/tobacco/smoking.html

Cannabis (drugs), Retrieved from http://en.wikipedia.org/wiki/

Marijuana

What is LSD, Retrieved from http://www.wisegeek.com/what-is-lsd.htm

Date Rape Drugs, Retrieved from http://www.medicinenet.com/script/main/art.asp?articlekey=21794

The National Drug Intelligence Center (NDIC), Retrieved from http://www.justice.gov/ndic/pubs6/6074/index.ht

Toxicologist Warning to Parents: Look for signs of K2 --'Fake Marijuana', Retrieved from http://www.sciencedaily.com/releases/2010/03/100303092405.htm

PCP, Retrieved from http://www.drugs.com/pcp.html
http://www.a1b2c3.com/drugs/pcp2.htm

Drug-Facilitated Sexual Assault (DFSA) Rohypnol, Retrieved from http://www.911rape.org/rape-drugs/rohypnol/what-is-rohypnol
http://www.usdej.gov/ndic/pubs6/6074/index.htm
http://www.ctclearinghouse.org

Teenagers smoking K2, Retrieved from http://drug-abuse.suite101.com/article.cfm/teenagers-smoking-k2-have-authorities-inccensed

What is LSD? Effects of Lysergic Acid Diethylamide, LSD Trip, Retrieved from http://www.healthhype.com/what-is-lsd-effects-of-lysergic-acid-diethylamide-lsd-trip-html

LSD Abuse and Effects, Retrieved from http://www.narconon.ca/LSD.htm

The National Drug Intelligence Center (NDIC), Retrieved from

http://www.justice.gov/ndic/pubs4/4260/index.htm
http://www.essortment.com/articles/lsd_10004.htm

Crack Abuse, Retrieved from http://www.drugrehab.net/2009/09/12/crack-abuse

The National Drug Intelligence Center (NDIC), Retrieved from http://www.justice.gov/ndic/pubs3/3978/index.htm

Addiction Search, Retrieved from http://www.addictionsearch.com/treatment_articles/crack-cocaine-addiction-abuse-and-treatment_28.html.

Side Effects of Cocaine, Retrieved from http://www.buzzle.com/articles/side-effects-of-cocaine.html

Cocaine Effects, Retrieved from http://www.cocaine-effects.com/

Cocaine Effects Symptoms, Retrieved from http://www.cocaine-effects.com/cocaine-abuse-symptoms.htm

Cocaine Side Effects, Retrieved from http://www.disabled-world.com/artman/publish/cocaine.shtml

Cocaine: Side Effects and Long-term Effects, Retrieved from http://mental-health.families.com/blog/cocaine-side-effects-and-long-term-effects

Cocaine Abuse, Retrieve http://www.emedicinehealth.com/cocaine_abuse/article_em.htm

Phencyclidine, Retrieve http://en.wikipedia.org/wiki/Phencyclidine

DrugFacts: Hallucinogens – LSD, Peyote, Psilocybin, and

PCP, Retrieved from http://www.drugabuse.gov/infofacts/hallucinogens.html

Dextromethorphan, Retrieved from http://www.drugs.com/dextromethorphan.html

DXM, WHAT THE BIG DEAL, Retrieved from http://www.dxmstories.com/facts.html
http://www.wikidoc.org/index.hph/2C-B-BZP
http://www.neurosoup.com/2c-b/
http://www.drug-abuse-support.com/special-k-drug.html

2C-B-BZP, Retrieve from http://en.wikipedia.org/wiki/2C-B-BZP

DXM Addiction, Abuse and Treatment, Retrieved from http://www.drugabusehelp.com/drugs/dxm/

Understanding the Teen Brain, Retrieved from https://www.urmc.rochester.edu/encyclopedia/content.aspx?ContentTypeID=1&ContentID=3051
http://www.drugwatch.ingo/a_DXM_analitical16.htm

https://www.justice.gov/archive/ndic/

Change Your Brain, Change Your Life (Before 25), Retrieved from https://www.psychologytoday.com/blog/the-author-speaks/201408/change-your-brain-change-your-life-25
http://www.dextroverse.org/whatis.html

Teen Deaths May Be From DXM in Cough Medicines, Retrieved from http://www.medicinenet.com/script/main/art.asp?articlekey=47278

What Is Scabies, Retrieved from http://www.wisegeek.com/what-is-scabies.html

Health NewsFlash, Retrieved from http://www.healthnewsflash.com/conditions/scabies.htm

What is Scabies, Retrieved from http://education.yahoo.com/reference/dictionary/entry/scabies

Smoking, Retrieved from http://adam.about.com/reports/000041_1.htm

About Sexually Transmitted Diseases, Retrieved from http://Kidshealth.org/teen/sexual_health/stds/std.html

What Is HPV, Retrieved from http://www.cdc.gov/hpv/WhatIsHPV.html

Scabies, Retrieved from http://www.stdsite.com/Scabies/Index.html

Scabies, Retrieved from http://www.aolhealth.com/conditions/scabies-major-1?
sem=1&ncid=AOLHTH00170000000017&s_kwcid=TC
%7c11093%7cw

http://www.righthealth.com/topic/Std_List/overview/
rh_uniquecontent?
fdid=rhuniquecontent_c7890eb73flc2b16acee0355e8d8c

http://www.alcoholism-information.com/
Side_Effects_of_Alcoholism.htm

Alcohol: Fast Facts, Retrieved from http://www.doitnow.org/pages/512.html
http://www.doitnow.org/wiki/Short-term_effects_of_alcohol

...ON YOUR HEALTH Alcohol, Retrieved from http://

www.med.unc.edu/alcohol/prevention/health.html

Alcohol, Retrieved from http://www.abovetheinfluence.com/facts/drugs-alcohol.aspx?id=search_properAlcohlol

Methamphetamine, Retrieved from http://en.wikipedia.org/wiki/Methamphetamine

Crystal Meth, Retrieved from http://www.druginfo.adf.org.au/druginfo/fact_sheets/ice_crystal_methamphetamine_hy.html

Crystal Meth Effects The Effects Of Crystal Meth And Methamphetamines, Retrieved from http://www.rehab-drug.net/crystal_meth_effects.html

Long Term Effects of Alcoholism, Retrieved from http://www.learn-about-alcoholism.com/long-term-effects-of-alcoholism.html

Side Effects of Alcoholism, Retrieved from http://www.alcoholism-information.com/Side_Effects_of_Alcoholism.html

Long-term effects of Alcohol, Retrieved from http://en.wikipedia.org/wiki/Long-term_effects_of_alcohol

The Not So Obvious Side Effects Of Alcoholism, Retrieved from http://ezinearticles.com/?The-Not-So-Obvious-Side-Effects-Of-Alcoholism&id=971766

Impact of Waxing on Skin, Retrieved from http://www.removinghair.co.uk/ImpactOfWaxing.html

Waxing, Retrieved from http://hairremoval.ygoy.com/2008/05/30/side-effects-of-waxing/

Tattoo, Retrieved from http://en.wikipedia.org/wiki/Tattoo

Think Before You Ink – Some Things to Know Before Getting a Tattoo, Retrieved from http://ezinearticles.com/?Think-Before-You-Ink---Some-Things-to-Know-Before-Getting-a-Tattoo&id=2322209

TATTOO'S Deadly Little Secret, Retrieved from http://www.av1611.org/tattoos/health.html

The Negative Effect of Body Art (Tattoos), Retrieved from http://www.r-go.ca/tattoo.htm

Tattoos: Understand Risks and Precautions, Retrieved from http://www.mayoclinic.com/health/tattoos-and-piercings/MC00020

Sexually Transmitted Diseases, Retrieved from http://stdsite.com?Molluscum/index.html

[Cytomegalovirus (CMV) Infection] What is Cytomegalovirus (CMV) Infections?, Retrieved from http://stdsite.com/CMV/index.html

[Scabies] What is Scabies?, Retrieved from http://stdsite.com/Scabies/index.html

What is Chancroid?, Retrieved from http://stdsite.com/Chancroid/index.html

Molluscum Contagiosum, Retrieved from http://www.youngwomenshealth.org/molluscum.html

Using a Fire Extinguisher, Retrieved from http://www.fire-extinguisher101.com/using.html

The ABC's of Portable Fire Extinguishers Selection, Use and

Maintenance

Use of Fire Extinguishers, Retrieved from http://www.ehow.com/how_4927373_use-fire-extinguishers.html

Chemicals in Cigarettes, Retrieved from http://www.quit-smoking-stop.com/harmful-chemicals-in-cigarettes.html

What Chemicals are in Cigarettes and Cigarette Smoke, Retrieved from http://quitsmoking.about.com/od/chemicalsinsmoke/a/chemicalshub.htm

Cigarettes Ingredients – Chemicals in Tobacco Smoke, Retrieved from http://www.tricountycessation.org/tobaccofacts/Cigarette-Ingredients.html

From the First to the Last Ash: The History, Economics & Hazards of Tobacco – Unit 1: History & Economics of Tobacco, Retrieved from http://www.healthliteracy.worlded.org/docs/tobacco/Unit1/1what_is.html

From the First to the Last Ash: The History, Economics & Hazards of Tobacco – Unit 2: Cigarette Advertising, Retrieved from http://www.healthliteracy.worlded.org/docs/tobacco/Unit2/1cigarett_adv.html

From the First to the Last Ash: The History, Economics & Hazards of Tobacco – Unit 3: Why People Smoke, Retrieved from http://www.healthliteracy.worlded.org/docs/tobacco/Unit3/1why_people_smoke.html

From the First to the Last Ash: The History, Economics & Hazards of Tobacco – Unit 4: The Dangers of Smoking Cigarettes for Smokers, Retrieved from http://www.healthliteracy.worlded.org/docs/tobacco/Unit4/1whats_in.html

Cigarettes' Deleterious Ingredients: "Toxic Tobacco Smoke" (TTS), Retrieved from http://medicolegal.tripod.com/

Lora McDuffie

toxicchemicals.htm

The Harmful Chemicals in Cigarettes, Retrieved from http://www.qualityhealth.com/cancer-articles/harmful-chemicals-cigarettes

Cancer Causing Chemicals in Cigarettes, Retrieved from http://www.healthcentral.com/copd/h/cancer-causing-chemicals-in-cigarettes.html

Smoking: What's In A Cigarette, Retrieved from http://pbskids.org/itsmylife/body/smoking/article3.html

Dangers of 69 Cancer Causing Chemicals in Cigarettes to Men, Women, and unborn Babies, Retrieved from http://www.ciggyfree.com/cigblog/2006/12/13/smoking-your-body/

-Cigarette Chemicals – Smoking Facts about the Added Chemicals in Cigarettes, Retrieved from http://www.smoking-facts-and-fiction.com/cigarette_chemicals.html#sthash.ZlJgFtt8.dpbs

Why do cigarettes have 4000 chemicals in them? Retrieved from http://ask.metafilter.com/57438/Why-do-cigarettes-have-4000-chemicals-in-them

Definition of Sexually transmitted disease, Retrieved from http://www.medterms.com/script/main/art.asp?articlekey=5472

SSL: Your Key to E-commerce Security, Retrieved from http://www.webopedia.com/DidYouKnow/Internet/2005/ssl.asp